KU-225-353

Contents

Appendices   107

W.O.M.H.T.
HILL CREST LIBRARY
QUINNEYS LANE
REDDITCH
WORCS

Going Paperless

A guide to computerisation in primary care

Nicola Shaw

Senior Research Associate
Centre for Health Services Research
University of Newcastle upon Tyne

Series Editor

Alan Gillies

Professor in Information Management
University of Central Lancashire

Foreword by

Glyn Hayes

Radcliffe Medical Press

Worcestershire Health Libraries

H05039

© 2001 Nicola Shaw

Radcliffe Medical Press Ltd
18 Marcham Road, Abingdon, Oxon OX14 1AA

All rights reserved. No part of this publication may be reproduced, stored in a retrieval system or transmitted, in any form or by any means, electronic, mechanical, photocopying, recording or otherwise without the prior permission of the copyright owner.

British Library Cataloguing in Publication Data

A catalogue record for this book is available from the British Library

ISBN 1 85775 519 7

Typeset by Action Publishing Technology, Gloucester
Printed and bound by TJ International Ltd, Padstow, Cornwall

Contents map

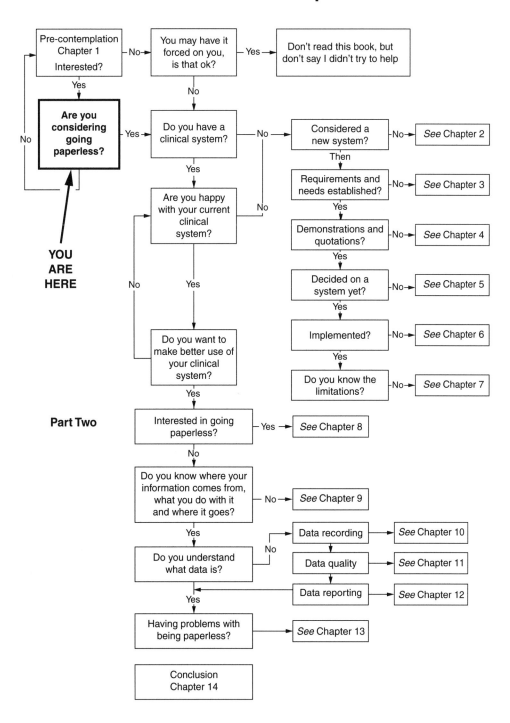

Foreword

Most books about primary care computing have been written by computer literate GPs. They thus have a great deal of experience of the practicalities of implementing and using computer systems in general medical practice. However, their knowledge is empirical and, although extremely valuable, their guidance is based on their own personal experience. They will be biased because of the particular systems they have used and by the type of practice they work in.

This book, by Dr Nikki Shaw, is written by a trained and experienced medical informatician. She understands medical concepts and the practice of medicine, and also the concepts and practice of information systems engineering. Her book is therefore a dispassionate and scientific analysis of the issues and problems facing those who need to develop the paperless practice. The result is a comprehensive and easy-to-read guide to one of the most pressing problems facing primary care.

Going paperless has been a major hurdle for many. It is the golden egg of medical information technology and many believe offers great promise for medical care. UK primary care computing leads the way in the world. It has a long history stretching back over 20 years. The systems have been developed, primarily by experienced GPs, into medical records that are more sophisticated and more comprehensive than those in other countries. The 'cradle to grave' NHS record, the need for lifelong total care and the registered list of patients have given us the opportunity to explore what computer systems can do. However, its full potential has been recognised by only the dedicated few, with most just using the computer for basic data collection. Now UK general practice has changed. The increasing bureaucracy, the need for accountability and the removal of the legal impediments mean that every practice now has to move towards fuller computerisation and the paperless practice.

The move from administrative computer use to full clinical systems requires changes in practice. It can damage the clinician–patient interaction that is so important in care. There are skills to be learnt about how to consult with a 'third party' in the consultation. Many are emotionally reliant on the old, inefficient manual records. It takes a lot to throw away years of experience and embrace new methods.

Yet the benefits are there to be had. As Dr Shaw says, the benefits of paperless practice are, with the exception of prescribing, not yet proven in formal scientific terms. Prescribing has been shown to be more effective with computer support. In other areas the evidence is growing. Better adherence to regular screening and guidelines of good practice have been shown to occur with the electronic medical record (EMR). The stumbling block has always been the dual use of paper and the EMR. Such practice means more work, transcription errors and inefficiency. The benefits only come when the paper is thrown away. As long as it is present clinicians will cling to the paper, no matter what benefits the EMR can bring. Once paperless they can develop the relevant skills to enhance their practice. Electronic information to guide the clinician and inform the patient improves care. Decision support can help when there is doubt about the correct way forwards. I believe the main advantage of the EMR is that it can make the known information about the patient more available. I remember being taught in medical school that the answer to the diagnosis of a patient with large notes always lay in those notes if one looked hard enough. Properly structured EMRs mean that the mass of data, buried in a paper record, can be seen, interrogated and, most importantly, used to prompt the clinician in a seamless and non-intrusive manner.

Although I feel that the main benefit of a paperless practice is improved individual patient care, the non-clinical benefits are also very important. Getting rid of paper means that all the data is available to run a practice, manage the health service and cope with medical audit. In these days of greater accountability clinicians have to be prepared to analyse what they do and to justify their actions to others. EMR data can provide continuous, almost effortless, audit of practice. No longer does examining standards of care mean trawling through cluttered paper notes. However it is vital that this new tool is used wisely. Clinicians need to understand the issues of data quality and how to understand the resulting information. This book deals with all these issues.

Such seamless data management also helps to run the practice more efficiently. Items of service (IOS) and other financial claims no longer mean filling hordes of forms and missing many actions that could have attracted a fee. The reports required by health authorities no longer mean hours of manual labour.

Yet, as Dr Shaw points out, none of this comes easy. Choosing the right system is the first step and it must be a system that provides facilities that will make clinicians want to use it. Too many systems in the past were just data collection tools, sucking data out of the user but giving nothing back. After choosing the right system comes learning to use it – training, training, training. It is not sufficient to learn which keys to press. Nor is it sufficient to just dump the system into the practice and expect to reap the benefits. It requires an understanding of its effect on patient care and practice management, and means learning about data and how to use it. One day these will be second nature but this book, comprehensive as it is, will significantly assist in developing the understanding and the skills.

I would echo one of Dr Shaw's statements. When you have done it, when all the hard work is in the past, when it no longer seems foreign but second nature, you will not want to go back!

Glyn M Hayes MBChB DRCOG FBCS
Family Physician
Chair, Health Informatics Co-ordinating Committee of the
British Computer Society
President, Primary Healthcare Specialist Group of the British Computer Society
glyn@conline.demon.co.uk
August 2001

Preface

'But the Emperor has nothing on!' said a little child.
The Emperor's New Clothes
Hans Christian Andersen 1805–75

Going paperless

Is the paperless practice a case of the Emperor's new clothes? Let's think about the story for a moment. The Emperor spends a lot of time and money having new clothes made and fitted. Eventually, they are finished and he dresses and walks down the street parading his new clothes. His friends and colleagues don't like to say anything. He has spent a lot of money after all. Then a small child speaks up. 'The Emperor has no clothes on.'

Now I am by no means suggesting that primary care system suppliers are selling us systems that are like the Emperor's new clothes – non-existent. However, I do think that for the vast majority of practices, most of the possible benefits of computerisation have been pretty much invisible.

When we buy a computer system we can see what we are getting for our money. Yet the more practices I work with the more I am convinced that we don't really get the most from all this investment. Our systems are under-used and we don't use them effectively.

Why?

I think the answer is simple:

We don't know how!

Admittedly, until the end of 2000 it was illegal for practices to be paperless, preventing us from getting every penny's worth of investment out of the systems. However, now that we can use the computer to record all of our medical records there are opportunities finally to reap the benefits of all the time and money that has been spent.

Conflict

Before we start to look at these let me just make one comment. I personally don't think that an electronic health record actually improves patient care for an individual patient during the consultation. As a patient, I would rather my GP talk to me than fiddle with some computer.

However, as a health informatician, I have worked for several years in primary care computerisation and know that there are huge benefits to be gained by practices and practice populations. In fact, as a member of a practice population I have to admit that my own health has been improved as a direct result of my GP effectively using their system for regular recalls.

So what is this book about?

This book is about just two things:

1 How to buy a primary care clinical system that does what you need it to do (Part One).
2 How to use your clinical system effectively (Part Two).

How to use this book

Now you may already have a clinical system that you are happy with, in which case you want to skip straight to Part Two. Alternatively, you might have no system at all or one that needs upgrading or replacing. In which case, Part One is for you.

The book is intended to be used as a guide. You can either read it from cover to cover or you can dip in and out of it, as you need.

To make it easier for you to pick up and put down at whim there are a number of common elements that run throughout the book to assist you in finding the bit you want.

A fairy story

As you read through the book you will find a fairy story. This story is about the members of the primary care team at the ABC Health Centre as they replace their clinical system and start to learn to use it effectively. ABC's full primary care team meet weekly. It is a fairy story!

I make no apologies for the stereotyping of the cast. My only comment is that, having worked with well over 200 practices during the last few years, it is amazing how often the stereotypes hold true.

Cast

Dr Jones	GP	Male, new partner to practice, young. IT literate.
Dr Thomas	GP	Female, recently returned to practice after maternity leave.
Dr Andrews	GP	Male, elderly, near retirement. Unsure of technology.
Katy Jackson	Nurse practitioner	Female, recently qualified to prescribe and undertake more chronic disease management. Frustrated by GPs' unwillingness to let her take on more disease management.
Alice Young	Practice nurse	Female, worked at the practice for 30 years, seen GPs come and go.
Tracy Clark	Receptionist	Female, young, just left school. Hates manual appointments system and pulling notes.
Mandy Brooks	Receptionist	Female, worked at the practice for 30 years, seen GPs come and go. Close friend of Alice.
Kim Timpson	Practice manager	Female, been at the practice 5 years. Uses PC a lot for management and accounts.

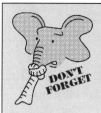

www link

This is a World Wide Web (www) link. It will tell you where you can find out more information on the Internet or NHSnet. All www addresses were correct at the time of press.

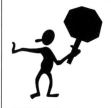

Resource materials

Nellie will show up now and again to let you know that there are relevant resource materials in the appendices that you might like to use. Copies of these are available for you to download from:

www.radcliffe-oxford.com/paperless

Caution

If this symbol is present, you are being cautioned or warned about something.

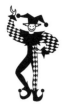

The jester

The jester will appear occasionally to remind you that you do need to keep your sense of humour when working with computers in primary care.

Key points

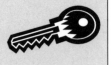

Each chapter will finish with a list of key points. Sometimes these will be things that you should do. At other times they might be things for you to think about.

Nicola Shaw
August 2001

Acknowledgements

Comments and editorial assistance were ably provided by a number of friends and colleagues whose assistance is gratefully acknowledged.

On a personal note – my thanks must go to my Mum, Mrs Pam Abraham, for reminding me that there is more to life than writing a book and to Molly, my dog, who was very clear that walks, cuddles and food always come first!

Contributions

A number of people and organisations helped to contribute towards this book.

Thanks are particularly due to Dr David Stables (EMIS), Dr Mike Robinson (IPS) and Dr Mike Bainbridge (Torex Health) who each gave their time for a detailed interview at very short notice.

Additionally, my thanks go to the Australian Commonwealth, Frank Quinlan and Professor Michael Kidd for granting permission for me to use some of the resource materials created by the Australian General Practice Computing Group (GPCG). My thanks to the Australian Commonwealth for funding this organisation. Long may it continue!

Likewise, my thanks to Sheila Teasdale for granting me permission to use some of the PRIMIS material and to Wendy Sutton-Pryce and Karen Wilson for providing copies at short notice.

Finally, the chapter maps were developed in collaboration with Dr David R Pepper, Associate Clinical Professor, University of California San Francisco.

Funding

This book was written in order to disseminate aspects of work undertaken by the author whilst funded as a National Health Service Executive (North West Region) Research and Development Post-Doctoral Training Fellow.

The support of the National Health Service Executive (North West Region) Research and Development department and Oldham Primary Care Group is therefore gratefully acknowledged.

This book is dedicated to my Grandfather, James Roberts Shaw (1921–1987)

In honour of his memory, and in recognition of his faith and belief in me, I took his name for my own in the summer of 2001.

Part One

Choosing a clinical system

Chapter 1: Pre-contemplation

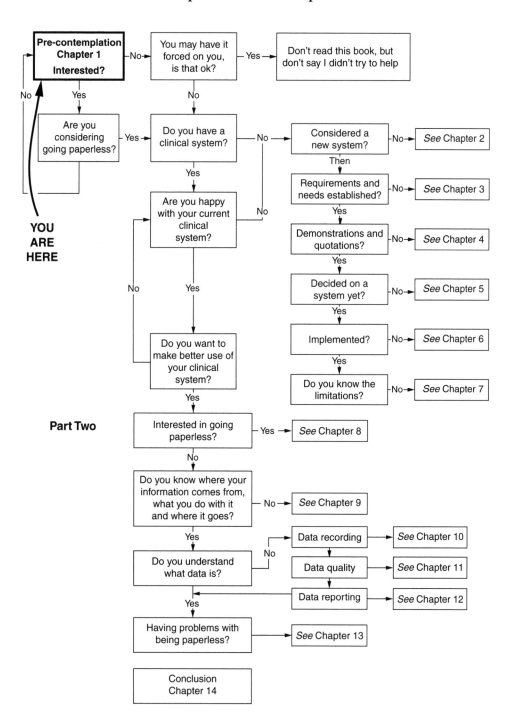

Pre-contemplation

Learning without thought is labour lost; thought without learning is perilous.
Confucius c.550–c.478 BC

Who should read this chapter?

There are three reasons for reading this chapter.

1 You don't have any form of an electronic patient record (EPR) system at the moment and require convincing that the hassle and expense are worth the benefits to be gained.
2 You have an EPR system but it is ineffectual and out of date and you need reminding as to why it seemed such a good idea at the time, before committing yourself to repeating that hassle and expense by changing your system.
3 You are simply reading this book from beginning to end in an effort to cure insomnia. Personally, I'd recommend a warm bath and a hot milky drink.

 ### Once upon a time ...

... there was a young GP, Dr Jones. Dr Jones had recently become a partner at the ABC Health Centre. The primary care team at the ABC Health Centre consists of a nurse practitioner, a practice nurse, two reception staff, a practice manager, Dr Thomas,

Dr Andrews and of course Dr Jones. Several members of the local community healthcare team also share their premises. Dr Jones' partners have little time for technology and while they do have an electronic patient record system, they make very little use of it.

Dr Jones is frustrated by the practice's use of paper records. When he was a GP registrar and medical student he worked in several practices that used electronic patient records and feels that there is a lot of benefit that their practice could gain from their use.

While he is happy to take on the management of information technology (IT) within the practice he recognises that first he needs to convince his partners that there are benefits from using an EPR system more effectively. However, he also knows that the system the practice currently has is very outdated and that considerable time and money may be required before these benefits can be gained.

During the weekly primary care team meeting he asks his colleagues what they think of their current EPR system. He is not surprised to find that they consider it useless and antiquated. After some discussion, he suggests that at the next team meeting they set aside some time to discuss this further.

This may or may not be a fairy story. However, it is true that there are many practices that either do not have an electronic patient record system or make little use of what they have. Therefore, let us consider Dr Jones' for a moment. At his next primary care team meeting, his general practitioner (GP) colleagues will undoubtedly air a long list of complaints about their current system. They will quote the amount of money it cost to purchase and to maintain. They will be emphatic that patients do not wish them to use it.

The electronic patient record – why?

How will Dr Jones persuade his colleagues that investing in their EPR is a good idea? Let's look at the evidence.

Managing and providing primary care-based patient care would be a simple prospect if patients:

- have *just* one medical condition
- never have medical emergencies
- never require secondary or tertiary care
- never travel beyond their home town
- never see more than one healthcare provider.

Unfortunately, this is not the case. Consequently, what has developed in primary care is the *cradle-to-grave (or sperm-to-worm) record.* This 'record' documents all ailments, treatments and interventions allowing each person reading that record to know what has gone before.

Historically, this 'document' has been paper-based and has followed a patient around the country each time they have registered with a new general practice. However, since the mid-1970s more and more GPs have opted to keep this record, to a greater or lesser extent, electronically. **Why?**

The carrot and stick

There are two reasons why GPs have opted to use EPR systems. The first is the carrot – personal (or practice)-based benefits. The second is the stick (sometimes cunningly disguised as a carrot) – key reforms and Government-led incentives.

Dr Jones prepared well for the primary care team meeting. He agreed that their current EPR had cost a lot of money and that there were issues that needed to be addressed. However, he also identified all the benefits that he had experienced when he had used an EPR in a 'paperless' practice. During the discussion, the reception staff said that they thought a computerised appointments system would be wonderful. Dr Thomas and Dr Andrews agreed that when they thought about it, they had actually gained financially from their limited use of their EPR through better management of items of service (IOS) claims. Dr Thomas also observed that there were far fewer calls from pharmacists clarifying prescriptions since they had started printing the prescriptions.

Being a tactful doctor, Dr Jones didn't suggest that the practice should consider going 'paperless' but instead suggested that he undertake a little research to find out what the practice needed, what was available and what the likely requirements were going to be on the practice from their primary care group (PCG) and health authority (HA). The primary care team were now interested in the potential while remaining sceptical. Dr Jones agreed to speak with their local PCG ICT manager and to report back at the meeting.

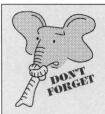

Appendix 1 provides a detailed and referenced list of benefits attributed to primary care EPRs.

Personal and practice-based benefits

- *Finance*: Practice income depends to a large extent on how well the practice list is managed. Typically EPRs maintain patient registers sorted alphabetically, by age and sex for screening/recall, for chronic diseases, and for repeat prescriptions. These age/sex and chronic disease registers can be used to call patients for fee-paying procedures thus increasing uptake and consequential financial payment.

- *Prescribing*: Computerised repeat prescribing has been shown to save a lot of time and effort and is believed to improve safety due to a combination of inbuilt contraindication alerts and the use of printed prescriptions as opposed to hand written, often illegible scripts.

- *Clinical governance*: The number of areas where practices are mandated to maintain chronic disease registers, minimum data sets and to report on the process of care is increasing. The use of an EPR is ideally suited to meet these requirements.

- *Clinical decision support tools*: The primary care team cannot be expected to know everything as the medical knowledge base is growing exponentially. The use of validated decision support tools; protocols, guidelines and templates can help to address this (e.g. drug interventions, healthcare maintenance).

- *Appointments*: Managing the appointments for the primary care team is a complex task. A number of rules have to be remembered (e.g. double-length appointments for smears). If a patient calls up having forgotten when their appointment is several pages of often illegible writing has to be read in an attempt to find the appropriate notation. Computerised appointments mean that such issues are easily addressed.

Government reforms and incentives

The move towards an EPR has been encouraged by a number of policy interventions alongside components of health service reforms[1] that have made it increasingly difficult to conduct primary care without the use of an electronic record.

1 *Items of service*: The 1967 GP Charter introduced additional payments for specific public health-related services such as contraception, cervical cytology and family planning. This led to a requirement for better recording of population-based health promotional activity for GPs.

2 *Reimbursement*: From 1989 a proportion of general practice information technology (IT) investment became directly remunerable. The computer reimbursement scheme currently offers partial recompense for the cost of computerisation conditional on the system implemented being RFA (*see* Chapter 2) accredited to the decreed level.

3 *Health promotion/financial incentives*: Contractual changes between GPs and the Government led to an element of pay being dependent on GPs reaching set targets for population-based care in the late 1980s/early 1990s. It was difficult to demonstrate reaching these targets without IT support.

4 *Purchaser/provider split*: April 1990 saw the commencement of GP fundholding. This invention by the Conservative Government allowed fundholding GPs to purchase care on behalf of their own patients. This resulted in the requirement for participating practices to introduce healthcare accounting packages within their systems. The cost of purchasing these systems was fully remunerable. However, in 1998 the new Labour Government announced its intention to replace fund-holding with compulsory commissioning. Consequently, from April 1999, commissioning has been carried out by primary care organisations (PCG/PCTs). Each commissioning organisation holds its own budget and decides what healthcare to purchase in accordance with its own population's needs. As a result of this there is an increasing emphasis on obtaining accurate and validated population-based data from general practices to ensure that services are commissioned appropriately.

5 *Health improvement targets*: Health improvement targets are set by national service frameworks (NSFs). GPs are required to report on their success at meeting these targets on a regular basis. It is difficult to demonstrate reaching these targets without IT support.

6 *Clinical governance*: Clinical governance was introduced to the NHS in the 1997 Government White Paper: *The New NHS: modern, dependable*.[2] Consequently, the quality of care as well as fiscal responsibility has for the first time been given equal weighting and priority within the NHS.

7 *Electronic health record (EHR)*: In 1998, *Information for Health*[3] set forth a vision for the National Health Service (NHS) of an EHR that would provide a single record of a person's contact with the NHS throughout their lifetime. In order to achieve this, the NHS needs to harness the information currently residing in primary care and consequently, in late 2000, the government removed the legal requirement for paper-based records allowing general practices to legitimately become paperless,[4] subject to their meeting conditions to be established by their local Health Authorities (HAs).

Key points

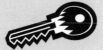

1 Managing and providing primary care-based patient care is not simple.

2 Evolution and development of 'cradle-to-grave' record.

3 Since the mid-1970s lots of GPs have started to use an electronic EPR system.

4 Benefits of EPRs are both carrots and sticks.

5 EPR systems can help practices to both eat the carrots and fend off the sticks.

Chapter 2: Contemplation

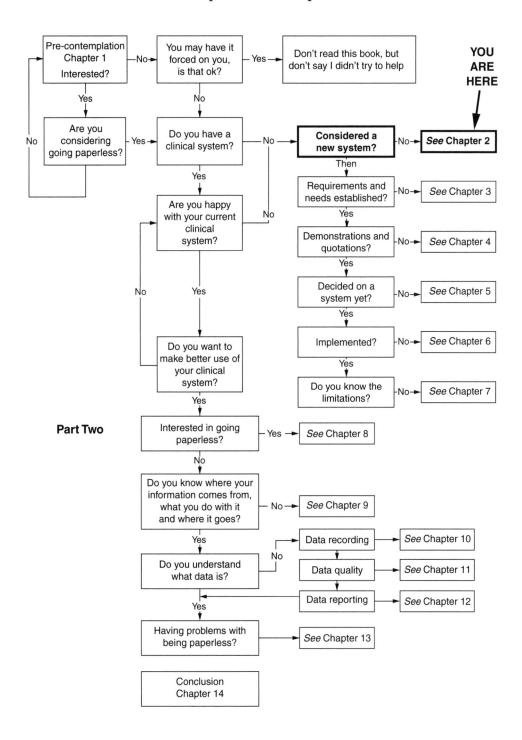

Contemplation

No man is an island, entire of itself.

Devotions John Donne 1571–1631

Who should read this chapter?

You have decided that an EPR is for you. However, before you rush out and purchase the first system that you come across there are a number of issues you need to consider. For after all, no GP or practice is an island.

Dr Jones contacted his local primary care organisation (PCO) and arranged for the ICT manager to visit the practice for a chat. He was aware that there was a lot of discussion going on at a national level about an EHR but hadn't paid much attention to the debate. He hoped that the manager would be able to bring him up to date.

The ICT manager provided a briefing for Dr Jones.

National policy

The Government has committed the NHS to developing and using an EHR across the NHS within the next four years.[3,5] An EHR is a record that provides a summary of a patient's healthcare history, wherever in the country they need care. This has a number of implications for primary care.

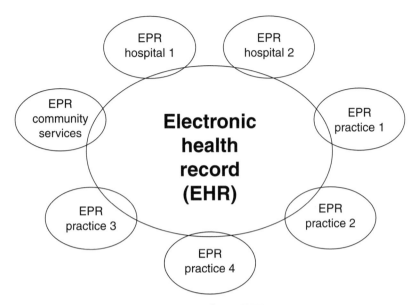

Diagram of an EHR.

The most important of these is that NHS management has recognised that there is a great deal of valuable data being recorded in primary care that must now be shared with other healthcare providers if this vision of an EHR is to be achieved. However, a great deal of discussion is needed as to how best this can be done.

Language barriers

If we look at the diagram of an EHR above, we can see that the EHR consists of bits of EPRs from different NHS organisations. The problem is that all these different EPRs talk different languages and have a lot of problems communicating with each other (e.g. chest pain, myocardial infarction (MI), heart attack). Even if we assume that either a common language or interpreters can be found, we still have another problem.

Ownership

That is *who owns the EHR*? Whose responsibility is it to create it, keep it up to date and protect it? If it is made up of lots of different bits that belong to lots of different organisations, who does the summary belong to? For the sake of argument, let's agree that all data created in the NHS belongs to the NHS (and we'll forget patient rights just for the minute).

How do we put it all together?

Even then we are still left with the problem as to whether data should be physically copied from each EPR into the overall EHR, or if the EHR should be a mechanism by which data in different EPRs can be viewed.

If you think that the data should be copied from each EHR, should it be *pushed* into the EPR with each individual organisation responsible for deciding what data is given into the EHR for others to share? Or should it be *pulled* from the EPR into the EHR, which makes the owner of the EHR responsible for deciding what data to extract from each of the different EPRs?

Due to these questions, and many others like them, there is no easy way of developing an NHS-wide EHR. Therefore, there are a number of different projects that are being developed in the NHS to try and find solutions to some of these issues.

WWW link   http://www.nhsia.nhs.uk/erdip

Implications for primary care

All this sounds very complicated and difficult but what difference does it make to whether or not Dr Jones advises his primary care team to look into the purchase of a new clinical system? The answer is that Dr Jones needs to find out what his local policy is in response to these national policies.

Throughout the country there are a groups of people developing and implementing local implementation strategies (LIS). These strategies are the ways that local groups of NHS organisations are agreeing how to work towards the vision of a NHS-wide EHR by 2004.

As is often the way in the NHS, it is unlikely that any two LIS are identical. These LIS teams should have considered the general practices within their region and there should be GP representation on the LIS team.

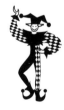

In addition to LIS teams local HAs and PPCGs and PCTs are directing local policy through health improvement programmes (HImPs) and more generally on computerisation in primary care. Ideally, as the LIS and HImP teams include representation from HAs and PCOs as well as secondary care trusts and community care, local policy should be identical whichever organisation you approach for information.

Local policy

Let's ignore secondary, community and tertiary care providers for a moment (in the good NHS tradition) and just look at how primary care can be affected by the decisions made by local policy.

Local policy makers can make a number of choices that radically change the way in which GPs have traditionally approached computerisation.

Centralisation

The first priority is for you to establish whether or not local policy is to continue to work with different systems or to replace all systems (or groups of systems) with one system. It is possible that an entirely new EHR system will be implemented throughout your area that would replace the need for individual systems. Whilst it is unlikely that GPs would be forced to change to this new system it may be *strongly* suggested that they would find it beneficial to do so.

One system for GPs

A decision that several PCOs have already implemented is to move all general practices within their area to just one system supplier. This has the advantage of bulk purchasing of software, hardware, maintenance and training. If you find that this is the case for your PCO, you will save yourself the time involved in looking at different systems and you will be offered incentives (e.g. a greater level of reimbursement) to change to the preferred system.

However, there are a number of problems with this approach.

- The first is that the PCO chosen system may not be the best suited to the particular way or working of your practice.
- Second, there is a concern about *'putting all your eggs in one basket'*. What happens if the supplier goes bust or simply cannot provide the level of post-sales support needed?

Additionally, one of the reasons PCOs are opting for one supplier for all their GP practices is to cut down on hardware costs and maintenance. Rather than having a server in each individual practice with individual maintenance costs, it is possible for practices to share a centralised server based in the PCO.

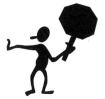
You *should* have reservations about this. As we discussed a little while ago (*see* Ownership) there is no consensus at the moment as to who owns the data in EPRs and the proposed EHR. Traditionally, GPs have seen the 'cradle-to-grave' record as their data and taken appropriate action to protect and secure it. Should this record be physically held out of the practice you would be

relying on non-practice staff to maintain and secure that server. Whilst accessing the data remotely is technically no more difficult than from within your own practice, would you even consider giving all your paper records to the PCO to look after?

Data mining

Another option that the local policy may have adopted is that of data mining. This option allows each organisation to continue to use the system they prefer relying on extracting data from these systems. For GP systems, there are now a number of ways that you can do this. Any financial reimbursement to practices for GP systems is only allowed if the system is RFA accredited.[6] RFA99 systems allow anonymous data to be electronically extracted from different GP systems in a common format, through the use of the MIQUEST[7] tool. Alternatively, modern systems have excellent searching and reporting features, which allow you to extract data direct from the systems themselves.

The PCO ICT manager and Dr Jones discussed the national development of EHRs for some time. She explained how the local LIS team were responding to national policy. Dr Jones was delighted to hear that, whilst the PCO had considered moving all of the practices to one clinical system, they had decided against this. Current local policy was to continue to allow practices to choose the system that best suited their practice.

Dr Jones then asked what the position was with regards to reimbursement. He knew that practices could apply for reimbursement against the cost of purchasing a clinical system. He also knew that there was a limit to what they could apply for and some rules on what was suitable for reimbursement.

The PCO IT manager explained that practices could be reimbursed for 50% of the purchase and maintenance costs as long as the system was RFA accredited to the most recent version.

Funding

To be eligible for reimbursement GPs must purchase a clinical system that is accredited as conforming to a standard specification as detailed by the requirements for accreditation (RFA) documentation. This ensures that basic functionality and system integrity are adhered to. There are alternative solutions available but your PCO is unlikely to be enthusiastic or supportive of your choosing these.

Requirements for accreditation

The current version of RFA is RFA99. Systems that satisfy all the mandatory requirements of RFA99, as outlined below, are awarded an accreditation status. RFA2001 is currently being revised and will be published imminently.

RFA99 contains the following main sections:

- *Core requirements* – privacy and security, year 2000 conformance, Read codes, NHS number, data standards and system configuration
- *Support and training* – support, documentation and training requirements
- *General functionality* – patient and practice administration, prescribing and dispensing and reports
- *Messaging and information exchange* – connection to NHSnet and electronic data interchange (EDI) requirements including HA/GP links and pathology report messages
- *Knowledge related functionality* – MIQUEST and PRODIGY
- *Strategic statement* – items that may be included in future versions.

WWW link

http://www.fhs.org.uk/gpservs/accred/rfa/

http://www.nhsia.nhs.uk/rfa/frhome.html

The PCO ICT manager provided Dr Jones with the contact details of the system suppliers that currently had systems with accredited RFA99 status.

Dr Jones felt that he now understood the wider context in which his practice's clinical system would have to work. He was aware that it would be essential for their system to be able to communicate with the local trust but that this should be possible for pathology and radiology reporting at least, due to the RFA specification.

He decided that the practice should now start to define what they wanted their clinical system to be able to do. At the next primary care team meeting he asked for some time on the agenda for the staff to talk about individual needs and wishes.

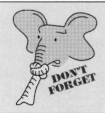

Appendix 2 provides you with a buyer's checklist.

Key points

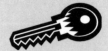

1 National policy will affect you – find out what it is!
2 Local policy will affect you – find out what it is!
3 Identify who is on your local LIS team and see if they can help you.
4 Find out what the local strategy is for computerisation in primary care from the LIS team, your HA and your PCO.
5 You must restrict your choices to RFA accredited systems if you want to be eligible for reimbursement.

Chapter 3: Requirements

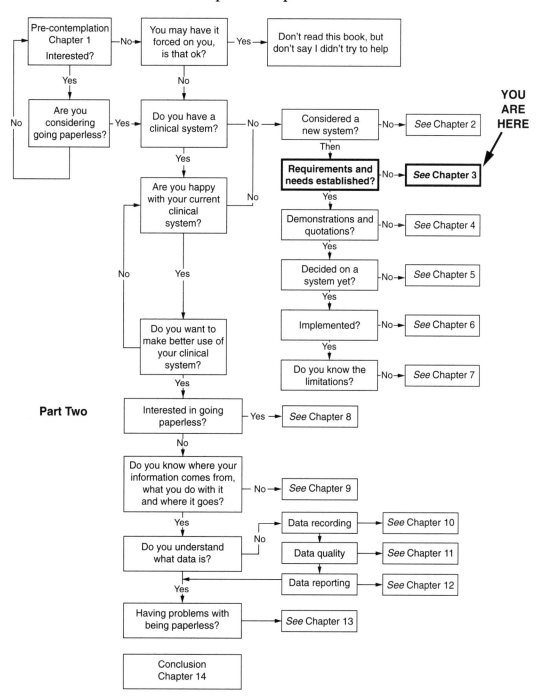

Requirements

From each according to his abilities, to each according to his needs.
Karl Heinrich Marx 1818–1883

Who should read this chapter?

You have decided that an EPR is for you and you have checked that there is nothing happening at a local policy level that affects what you can do.

However, before you rush out and purchase the first system that you come across you need to decide what you want the system to do, i.e. what your requirements are. It may surprise you to know that most people have a pretty woolly idea of what they want and need from their computer systems. It may also surprise you to know that time spent deciding this at the beginning will repay itself many times over.

At the next primary care team meeting Dr Jones asked everybody to list what they wanted the system to do. They came up with some ideas but after a short while they ran out of steam.

Alice (practice nurse) pointed out that they didn't actually know what was possible.

Identifying your requirements

You can actually decide your system requirements in just five steps. The outcome is known as a requirements specification.

A good requirements specification provides a detailed list of functions that you and your staff wish to achieve with your system. The specification should be used as a checklist for suppliers and helps you in working out which system best meets your specific needs. It should be reviewed and revised frequently until you are completely satisfied with it.

Step 1: identification of functions (needs assessment)

Dr Jones had the right idea in asking the staff what they wanted but Alice also had a good point. As the system they had been using was old and out of date they had never really appreciated what was possible. There are a number of ways that Dr Jones could help the practice team to list their needs.

1　They could each consider the grid of functional areas listed below and complete the grid for their own areas of concern. These grids could then be joined together to make one master grid. (A number of examples are provided to get you started.)
2　They could meet as a team and talk through what happens to a patient in a specific case scenario. To do this they would need to think about questions such as: what information is collected when, by whom and how is it then used? (This activity will at least identify specific patient registration, appointments, consultation, prescribing and billing functions that staff undertake.)
3　Dr Jones could arrange for the practice team to visit organisations already using EPRs and if possible to shadow somebody who undertakes a role similar to their own.

Appendix 3 provides you with details of GPIMM, which is a tool that may help you identify your needs.

Grid of functional areas

	Clinical	*Non-clinical*
Secretarial	Reminders	Patient registration Appointments
Business	Referrals	Billing Purchasing Salaries
Communications	External communication (pathology, radiology results)	Internal messaging
Audit	Assuring optimum treatment and follow-up	Re-call
Consultation	EHR (SOAP notes) Patient handouts Prescribing (acute and repeat)	
Decision support	Drug interactions Allergies Contraindications Protocols Integrated care pathways	

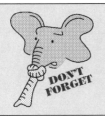

Appendix 4 is a list of questions you could ask your staff about your current system to prompt discussion.

Step 2: identification of issues

Having created a long list of needs (or functions). There are a number of issues that you will also need to address as part of your system requirements. You may be able to identify a system that meets every single one of your functional requirements. However, if the technical support and maintenance provided is very poor I can assure you this will prove meaningless.

All staff should be asked to consider what they need in terms of:

- technical support (e.g. speed, level of support, telephone versus personal)
- future proofing (e.g. frequency of maintenance and upgrades)
- methods of data entry (e.g. keyboard, mouse, voice recognition, etc.).

Step 3: identify resources

It is necessary to identify not only financial resources available but also physical requirements and staff skills (training requirements). Two of the biggest hurdles to a paperless practice are that:

- many current healthcare providers cannot type
- some older premises cannot support a computerised network.

The best method of identifying these requirements is to arrange a programme of:

- system demonstrations
- visits to organisations using the systems you are interested in
- asking friends and colleagues about their experiences
- visits to exhibitions to see suppliers' demonstrations
- asking local experts.

This will help to identify not only training requirements and physical resources but also the financial extras that are hidden at the point of purchase and only reveal themselves at a later date.

You may like to go further and carry out a formal training needs analysis.

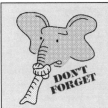

Appendix 3 contains details of a tool called TNAMM, which you may like to use to carry out a formal training needs analysis.

Step 4: prioritise

Now that you have a long, detailed list of functions and requirements you need to agree as a team, the functions that you *really* need, which are your priorities and those that you would like but that you wouldn't sell your grandmother to have, which form a secondary list.

Step 5: context

You have now written a very detailed, prioritised requirements specification. There is one more thing to do before you start using this as a basis for working out which system best meets your needs. You must look at the specification as a whole. It is very easy to get so ingrained in the detail of individual functions that you forget that you are working within a national framework. All specifications must contain a requirement for the system to meet:

- national medico-legal standards (especially regarding security and confidentiality)
- local and national requirements for data recording.

 Dr Jones decided to arrange visits to local practices that were using clinical systems, and in fact regarded themselves as 'paperless'. He gave each member of the practice team a copy of the grid and asked them to think about what they would like the system to do for them in each of these areas. He also asked them to think about what it could do for their colleagues.

After they had all done this, they met as a primary care team again. At this meeting Dr Jones talked through a case scenario with them and they each checked that each time they wanted to record or know something about the patient this was noted in their grid as a requirement.

Dr Jones then filled in a huge grid, with everybody's needs and wishes.

Kim (practice manager) had spent a lot of time talking to the practice managers in the practices they had visited about the other issues they should consider. She now had a very detailed list of what she required in terms of support and maintenance.

Dr Andrews was still unsure about this typing malarkey, He was sure it would annoy him when he was with a patient. However, he quite liked the idea of voice recognition and was going to go back and visit his friend to see this working again. Also, another colleague had suggested that he take a short typing course at the local college. Apparently the typing course was free, for just two hours a week for six weeks and his friend (who was older than he was!) said he wouldn't be without his clinical system now and that the patients actually liked him using the computer as they could see what he was saying about them.

Dr Jones added Kim's requirements and Dr Andrew's interest in voice recognition to the grid. They then prioritised each of the needs with a star if they considered it essential and a triangle if it would be nice but they could do without it.

Dr Jones then agreed to take this prioritised list and discuss it with the PCO ICT manager to check that they had not forgotten any medico-legal issues or local and national requirements. The PCO ICT manager thought the list was excellent and just reminded Dr Jones to ensure that they had a look at PRODIGY and MIQUEST when they started to look at demonstrations.

Dr Jones was unsure what these were but didn't like to ask so he just agreed.

Dr Jones was then ready to request demonstrations and quotations.

Key points

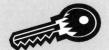

1 Be as detailed as you can when listing your needs.
2 Include all members of the primary care team when deciding what your needs are.
3 Think about your needs for system support as well as what you want the system to do.
4 List your available resources, both financial and staff.
5 Prioritise!
6 Don't forget the legal requirements!
7 If you don't understand something – ask!

Chapter 4: Demonstrations and quotations

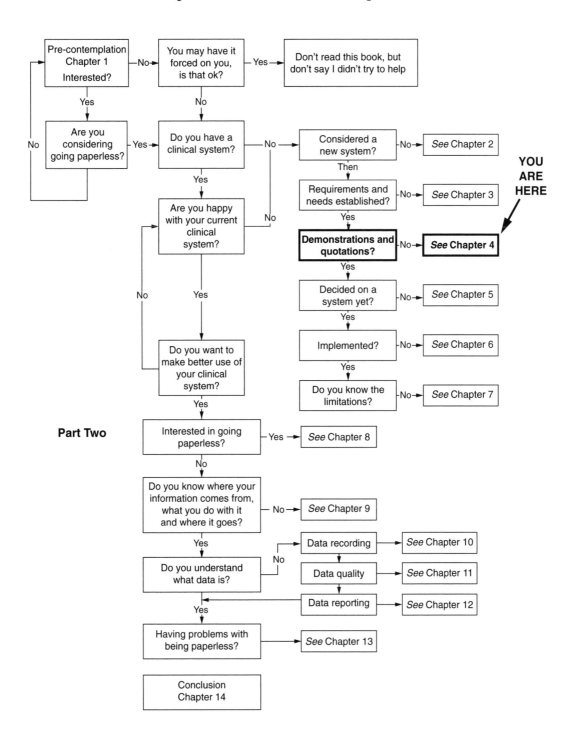

Demonstrations and quotations

Where large sums of money are concerned, it is advisable to trust nobody.
Agatha Christie 1891–1975

Who should read this chapter?

You have decided that an EPR is for you and you have checked that there is nothing happening at a local or national policy level that affects what you do. You also have a prioritised list of all the things an EPR *must* do for your primary care team and another list of the things you would like it to do.

 The PCO ICT manager gave Dr Jones contact details for the major EPR systems suppliers for GPs. He was surprised to find that there were over 20 different system suppliers in England but that just three suppliers dominated 85% of the market. Dr Jones used the Internet to check which of these suppliers systems were currently RFA accredited to the most recent version.

Dr Jones completed the outline of a *request for a proposal* given to him by his PCO ICT. He then sent copies of this to each of the three major suppliers. He asked them to:

- arrange to visit the practice and demonstrate their system

- provide him with contact details for local practices where he could go and see the system in practice

- address his list of requirements and list which bits they could do and which bits they couldn't.

Dr Jones rang the PCO ICT manager and asked her if she would like to attend the demonstrations. She said that she would love to and reminded him that he should only request demonstrations of 'third generation systems'. Dr Jones wasn't sure what she meant by this and asked her to explain.

She explained that traditionally the majority of EPR clinical systems in primary care are text based. This was because they were written in older languages. However, in the last few years system suppliers have been bringing their systems up to date so that they can make use of Windows®. Third generation systems simply mean that they are fully written in Windows®, rather than being text-based with a Windows® interface.

Dr Jones wasn't sure that he understood this but did know that he wanted the system to use Windows®, as he was used to that. His kids had a PC at home and that used Windows®.

Review available products

There are over 20 EPR system suppliers in the UK.[8] However, just three suppliers dominate 85% of the market: EMIS, In Practice Systems and Torex Health.[9]

EMIS

EMIS has two systems. A text-based system called EMIS LV and a Windows®-based system (released Spring 2001) called EMIS GV.

In Practice Systems (IPS)

IPS also sells two systems. Like EMIS LV and GV, Vamp Medical is text-based, whilst Vision is Windows®-based.

Torex Health

Torex Health maintain and sell many systems. However, they have three systems that fit Dr Jones's criteria of being RFA accredited and Windows®-based: Torex Premier, Visual Phenix and Torex System 6000.

Torex have stated that they will be merging Torex Premier and System 6000 into one system within the next two years (by about 2003). They have stated that it will not matter which of these systems practices use as the new system will be able to upgrade from either.

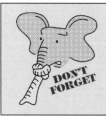

Appendix 5 will give you a brief description of EMIS, In Practice Systems and Torex Health.

Request for a proposal (RFPs)

When you contact the suppliers it is best if you can be as detailed as possible. A request for a proposal or RFP asks suppliers to look at your list of needs and identify whether their system meets all of them or not.[10] It also asks them to provide you with an estimated cost.

Suggested content of a RFP

Covering statement
This first section should give the supplier details of who they should contact at the practice and any deadline you have chosen for the proposal to be sent to you. It should also ask the supplier to arrange to visit your practice and demonstrate their system. You can also ask for contact details of local practices where you can go and see their system in practice.

Description of the practice
You need to provide a broad overview of your practice. You must include the number of staff and GPs, whether you have a branch surgery, a description of the buildings and any existing systems.

Requirements specification
This is when you give the supplier that long detailed list of needs you agreed. Remember to give them the prioritised and latest version.

Method of evaluation
You may choose to tell the suppliers what you will be assessing them on. It may well be that particular functions, ease of use, adequate training or price are far more important to you than anything else.

Details required
Don't forget to include a list of any specific questions you want the supplier to answer. For example, you may like to ask about:

• software required (number of licences)
• hardware required (computers, wiring, furniture)

- system documentation (manuals for system use and maintenance)
- maintenance and ongoing costs (specifics of what is covered and what isn't – including response times – and what may have to be purchased later)
- training (how much, how long will it take, on the job or off-site, classroom or demonstrations?)
- implementation (timetable of implementation process)
- ongoing support (arrangements for troubleshooting and advanced training, 24/7 availability?)

Cost
Be very precise about how you want the costs to be detailed. If you insist that the suppliers list each purchase component separately it will make it easier for you to compare proposals from different suppliers. Do ask for as much detail as possible.

Required conditions of purchase
Don't forget that you are potentially spending a lot of money with these suppliers. Give them details of any requirements you have for the system to be fully functional and working before you will agree final payments.

Suggested configuration
Give the supplier a description of what you think are the most likely requirements. Include the number of users and the main tasks they will do. This should allow suppliers to propose alternative configurations or amendments if necessary.

Source: GPCG (1999) *Buying Computer Systems For General Practice.* Version 1.2, June, pp 18–19. © Commonwealth of Australia, 1999

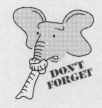

Appendix 6 provides a copy of the suggested content of a request for a proposal.

Demonstrations

When the suppliers contacted the practice, Dr Jones arranged for them to demonstrate their system, for an hour, to the entire primary care team. Before the supplier arrived, Dr Jones gave each member of the team a copy of the list of needs they had agreed as a reminder.

Ideally, you would ask all the suppliers to set up demonstrations side by side so that you can compare one system with the other more easily. It is unlikely that you will find suppliers willing to do this. However, if the timing is right for you there is a way of doing this.

The British Computer Society (in conjunction with the *British Journal of Healthcare Computing and Information Management*) organises an annual conference every Spring called Healthcare Computing. This is usually held in March and all the major system suppliers attend and exhibit their systems. While they rarely choose to occupy exhibition stands that are side by side they are at least in one place. This means that it is possible for you to ask the same question of all the systems suppliers and see the answer for yourself.

Alternatively, if March isn't convenient for you there is a smaller conference run by the British Computer Society Primary Health Care Specialist Group (BCS PHCSG) in June/July each year. While the exhibition is much, much smaller than that at Healthcare Computing EMIS, IPS and Torex usually exhibit.

WWW link	http://www.phcsg.org.uk/ http://www.healthcare-computing.co.uk

If neither of these are suitable, ask your PCO or HA ICT manager for other conference and exhibition details. There are other events that run throughout the year that the suppliers will attend and exhibit at.

Practice visits

Some of the primary care team had visited other practices to look at their systems when they had been trying to write a list of their needs. However, as they had each visited practices where they knew colleagues or had friends, they had seen a variety of systems and were not always sure exactly which system they had seen.

Using the details given to him by the suppliers, Dr Jones arranged for the primary care team to visit three local practices. One practice was using EMIS GV, one was using IPS Vamp Vision and the third was using System 6000. Dr Jones also visited a practice using Torex Premiere.

While visiting the practices each member of the primary care team concentrated on looking at the parts of the system that they would mainly be using:

- Doctors Andrews, Thomas and Jones looked at the medical record and prescribing

- Katy and Alice (practice nurse and nurse practitioner) looked at the way the systems manage chronic disease and new patient checks

- Tracy and Mandy (reception) looked at the appointments system and repeat prescribing

- Kim (practice manager) was specifically interested in the way the systems managed items of service links and registration.

They also all looked at reporting and how the system supported the creation and maintenance of chronic disease registers.

The more they looked at the systems, the more Mandy became worried. She could see that if all the doctors started to use an EPR system to record their medical notes they wouldn't need her to file paper notes any more and neither would she be needed to pull notes for each surgery.

Dr Jones noticed that Mandy was worried and took a minute or two to reassure all the staff that their jobs were not at risk. However, he did say that this was an opportunity for them to re-think how the practice works and how their jobs might change as a result.

Mandy was a little less worried by this but still unsure that she really wanted her job to change. She liked it.

Dr Andrews also grew more unsure about the idea of using an EPR in his consultations. He had been back to see his friend who was using voice recognition. He had been horrified to find out how many hours his friend had had to spend training the software to understand his voice. He was now really unsure that he wanted to use an EPR with his patients. Yet he could see how much more efficient it would be for the practice and he loved the idea of being able to check that all his patients who had had an MI were on aspirin.

Those awkward questions you need to ask!

When you visit your friends and colleagues ask them what questions they wish they had asked. You may find that there are specific areas that cause problems.

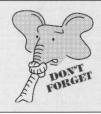

Appendix 7 is a list of questions you could ask the suppliers.

Data conversion

The most common problem for practices when they are changing from one system to another is data conversion or transfer. The problem is that the way data is stored is very different in different systems and suppliers have to do a lot of work to transfer data from your old system to your new one. They have a lot of experience with this and it is much easier than it used to be. However, it does still seem to be the biggest cause of hassle and complaints. If you need to have data converted, be very detailed when you discuss this with suppliers. Contact a practice that has changed from the same system that you have been using and ask them about their experiences.

If you have been using your existing system for some time and either haven't

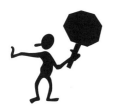

used it to record much clinical information or you know the data quality is very poor (*see* Chapter 10) you should consider writing it off.

Getting your data right takes a lot of work. You may find it easier to start with a fresh slate and simply have your patient list downloaded from Exeter and just have your prescribing and disease registers converted to the new system.

Key points

1 Understand the jargon or find somebody who does.
2 Talk to your friends and colleagues – ask about experiences, specifically any difficulties.
3 Visit practices, see systems in real use, ask about post sales support and maintenance.
4 Use a request for a proposal to ask for information from the suppliers. Using a standard request will make it easier for you to compare the proposals you get later on.
5 Finance – don't forget to include training and support as well as hardware and software.
6 Insist on presentations/demonstrations from suppliers being tailored to your interests and requirements.

7 Find out from your colleagues and friends *'those awkward questions'* they wish they had asked – and ask them!

8 Remember that suggestions from suppliers may change your requirements.

9 If suppliers do not assist in decisions and discussions, avoid them!

10 Put everything in writing!

Chapter 5: The decision

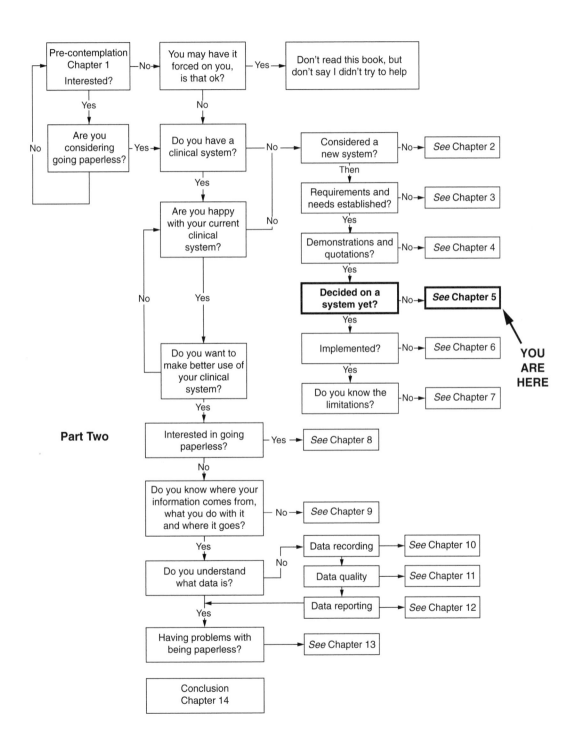

The decision

Who shall decide when doctors disagree?
Moral Essays III.1
Alexander Pope 1688–1744

Who should read this chapter?

You have decided that an EPR system is for you. You have checked that there is nothing happening at a local or national policy level that affects what you do. You have had system demonstrations and visited practices using systems live. You have received proposals in response to your request from the suppliers.

All three of the major system suppliers visited the practice and demonstrated their systems. Dr Jones has now received proposals from all of them.

At the next primary care team meeting Dr Jones asked all the staff to say what they thought about each system. He asked them to think specifically about the bits of the system that they had looked at in detail – the parts that they would be using themselves.

It was quite clear from this discussion that the GPs liked one of the systems more than the others. Unfortunately, it was just as clear that the rest of the practice staff preferred a different system. Even after a lengthy discussion about the two systems the team could not agree on one system.

Eventually, the PCT agreed that Dr Jones would review the proposals and make a decision. The GPs agreed that if Dr Jones couldn't choose between the two systems after reviewing the proposals the final decision would be based on expected costs over a five-year period.

Review proposals and costs

Now that you have full proposals from the suppliers you need to compare them against each other and also against your requirements specification. Even though you asked the suppliers to do this you *must* check for yourself. Whilst it can be very difficult to compare one system proposal with another in terms of the hardware and software, you should be able to compare each against your list of needs and wishes.

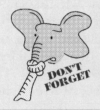

Appendix 8 is a checklist that you can use to compare hardware specifications from different proposals.

Dr Jones was very thankful that he had asked all the suppliers to provide their proposals in the same format as it made it easier to compare them. However, they still seemed to contain a lot of jargon so he contacted the PCO ICT manager who arranged to spend a couple of hours with him discussing the proposals and explaining the jargon where needed.

Clarification

If there is anything that you are unsure of, ask! Do not assume anything. If the suppliers have not been explicit about the number of days training or the expected response time for help, insist that they give you this information.

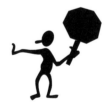

Costs

When comparing costs be very careful to check that you are comparing like with like. The best way of doing this is to ask the suppliers to give you total costs over a five-year period, to include all maintenance, support and training charges as well as initial purchase and installation costs.

Making the decision

At the end of the day it is often not easy to make a decision between available systems. It is rare that one system can be exactly what an entire primary care team wants. In reality, it is common for the final decision to be based on cost or on GP preference. If you can't decide there are a number of things you can do to help you make up your mind.

- *Negotiate*: Talk to the suppliers and ask them about the things you like in their competitors' systems. You may find that they can actually provide the same functions but hadn't made as much of them as the other supplier. Costs may be flexible if there is more than one practice buying a system at the same time so talk to your PCO and check that there aren't any other practices that are looking to buy a new system at the same time as you.
- *Dictate*: Make the decision based on your own personal preference or that of the GPs. At the end of the day a large proportion of the costs are going to come from the GP's pocket so why shouldn't their opinion be the one that counts?
- *Benevolence*: Make the decision based on practice staff's personal preference. It may be that you want the staff to make much more use of the system. Choosing the system that they prefer will gain you 'brownie points' in their eyes and make it easier for you to expect them to use it.
- *Draw lots*: Put the names in a hat and draw lots. Choose the system that you draw first. This is not recommended. (It would be rather distressing if you have read this far in the book and feel that this is the only way of making the decision.)

Dr Jones found that even after he had reviewed the proposals, the decision was still between the two systems that the primary care team had been discussing. He contacted the suppliers again and asked them about the specific features that the primary care team had liked in their competitor's systems. He found that one of the systems could do everything that they liked in the other system. This almost made the decision for him but just to make sure he compared expected costs over a five-year period. He found that there was very little difference. His final decision was for the system that the practice staff liked best.

Documenting agreements

Once you have decided which system you want contact all the suppliers you have been dealing with and let them know your decision. It is common for either the HA or the PCO to take a more active role at this point as you now need to get into the muddy area of contracts and legal agreements.

Dr Jones spoke to the primary care team and let them know the decision. The practice staff were very happy. Dr Andrews and Dr Thomas agreed with his decision once he had assured them that the system he had chosen could do all the things they liked in the other system.

Dr Jones then wrote to all three suppliers to let them know his decision. He also rang the PCO ICT manager to let her know their decision. She offered to assist with the contracts and implementation arrangements. Dr Jones accepted her offer readily.

Contracts

Regardless of whether or not the PCO or HA take the lead on the contractual and legal parts of purchasing a system you must check that you are happy with the contract before it is signed and finally agreed. There are a number of things you should look for specifically:[11]

Contract checklist

1 Does the contract include a clear, fixed price for the completed work?
2 Does the contract include detailed specifications of the work that is to be completed?
3 Does the contract include a detailed timetable for the completion of all work, including both installation and training and data conversion/transfer?
4 Does the contract include a detailed schedule of payments based on the timetable for the completed work? Will you have adequate opportunity to check the completed work?
5 Does the contract include the provision of adequate documentation for the new system?
6 Does your ongoing service agreement include arrangements for disaster recovery? Does this include a guaranteed response time if you have problems?
7 Does the contract include provision for you to access the software source code if your software supplier goes out of business?
8 Does your contract guarantee upgrades for a specified period?
9 Are any special arrangements of verbal agreements made between you and the supplier included in the written contract?

Source: GPCG (1999) *Buying Computer Systems For General Practice.* Version 1.2, June, p. 23.
© Commonwealth of Australia, 1999

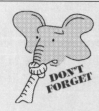

Appendix 9 contains a full copy of the GPCG contract checklist.

Key points

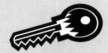

1 Check supplier proposals against your requirements specification. If the supplier does not explicitly state whether or not the system can meet the needs, ask!
2 If you don't understand, ask and keep on asking until it is explained in a way that you do understand.
3 Try and ensure you compare like with like as much as possible.
4 Deciding between the different systems can be very difficult.
5 Make a decision and tell everybody what that decision is.
6 Get *everything* in writing.
7 Check the details of your contract.

Chapter 6: Implementation

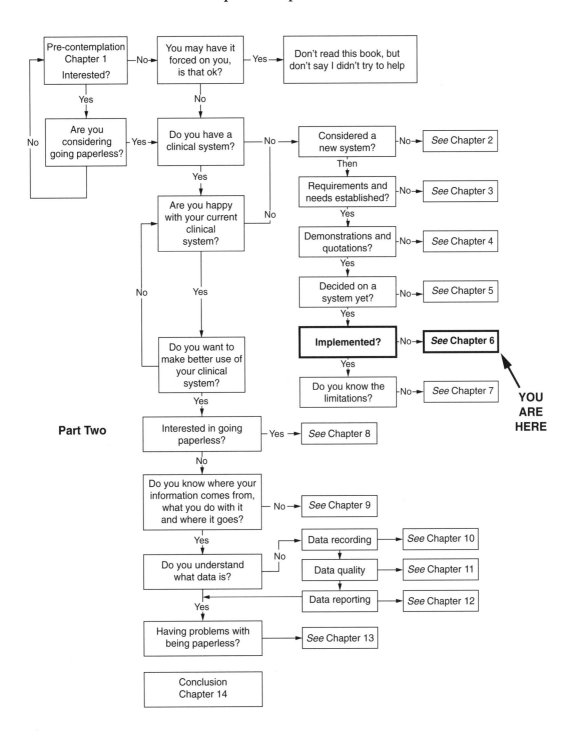

Implementation

If you do what you have always done, you'll get what you've always gotten.

Anon

Who should read this chapter?

You have decided that an EPR is for you and have gone through a full review process before deciding on the system you have agreed to buy.

> The PCO ICT manager, with Dr Jones, negotiated with the supplier and agreed a plan of implementation.

Develop plan of implementation

Time spent on planning the implementation of your new system is time well spent
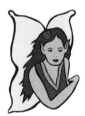 as the more you think about and consider before you go ahead, the fewer problems you will have when actual implementation starts. Your supplier should develop the implementation plan, with your assistance. If they don't, think again about your choice of system supplier.

Practice preparations

You may need to make physical changes to your premises. This may be as simple as rearranging some of the furniture or as complex as having false floors and ceilings put in to accommodate the network wiring. If you have had a system before, think about all those times when you have thought *'wouldn't it be better if ...'* and do what you can to check that these issues are thought about. It may be that having an additional printer would make life much easier or putting the computer in a different corner of the room would stop the sun from shining on the screen during afternoon surgeries.

The triad

At this point it is very important that you think about how the computer affects your relationship with the patient during a consultation. It has been suggested that it works best if the EPR system physically forms a triangle with the patient and the healthcare provider so that both the patient and the healthcare provider can see the screen.

From what I have seen, this triangle does work well *but* only once the healthcare provider is fully familiar with the EPR and comfortable with typing in front of their patient.

Staff preparations

It is essential that all staff know what is to happen and when it will happen. Additionally, this is an ideal time to look at the way the practice works and how staff roles will and could change within the practice.

There are also a number of new tasks that will need to be given to people. For example, who will:

- do the backups and backup testing
- manage routine system maintenance
- manage virus protection updates?

Do remember that it will take a *lot* of time for all the staff to get used to the new ways of working. Especially, if they have not used an EPR system before.

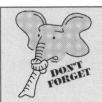

Appendix 3 contains details of GPIMM and TNAMM, which are tools that can be used together to help you plan your training needs and consider how staff roles will change as you develop use of your EPR system.

Dr Jones remembered that Mandy had been very worried about how her job would be affected by the new system. He also knew that Dr Andrews was very uncertain about using the computer when he had a patient with him.

While the entire primary care team had agreed to go ahead with buying the new system he wanted to make the implementation as painless for the practice as he could. He suggested that he would meet with his GP colleagues, then the nurses, and then the reception staff, to discuss how their roles might change.

Dr Andrews and Dr Thomas had very mixed feelings about the new system. It was a *lot* of money. It was just starting to sink in that they had a lot to learn before they would really see any benefits.

The doctors agreed that they did want to stop using paper notes. However, Dr Thomas was worried that this meant that she wouldn't have any of the paper-based information about a patient for use in the surgery. Dr Jones explained that he had arranged for the system supplier to convert all the data from their old system to their new system. This meant that all their prescribing and demographic information would be available to them. Additionally, he explained that it was possible for them to have all their paper-based registers entered on the system if they wished but that this would cost a little more. After some discussion, the doctors agreed that they wanted this information on the system. They also agreed that they really didn't want to run both a computerised and paper-based system so they would see if they could manage without pulling the paper-based notes. Of course, the paper notes would be there if they needed them.

Dr Andrews was still uncertain about using the computer itself. While Dr Thomas and Dr Jones had both used computers themselves and were quite good at typing, Dr Andrews felt as though he was 'all thumbs'. He had looked at voice recognition but didn't really like it. Dr Jones explained that the system-specific training would help and that they could get the system configured to make it easier for Dr Andrews. He explained that Dr Andrews would not need to use the mouse unless he wanted to and that most things could be entered quite quickly with just a few keystrokes. They agreed to restrict the number of available appointments for all the doctors for the first four weeks and for Dr Andrews for the first eight weeks after installation to give the doctors a little more time to get used to using the system during the consultation.

The doctors also agreed that Katy (nurse practitioner) and Alice (practice nurse) would be primarily responsible for chronic disease management. They had established chronic disease clinics some time ago and had been itching to take on more responsibility.

Katy and Alice were delighted to hear this when Dr Jones met with them. Katy immediately started to plan what else they could do. Dr Jones left them discussing something to do with templates and protocols.

Dr Jones then met with Tracy and Mandy (receptionists). They were quite worried because a lot of their time was currently spent pulling and filing notes and this wouldn't be needed anymore. However, when they thought about what their colleagues were doing at the practices they had visited they realised that there would be a lot of other things for them to do. After discussion, Tracy agreed to take on repeat prescriptions whilst Mandy was looking forward to managing appointments using the computerised system.

Finally, Dr Jones took a cup of tea in to see Kim (practice manager). She seemed to have been very quiet throughout all of this and he was a little worried that she was unhappy about it all. She was quick to reassure him that she was very pleased about it but that her workload was very high at the moment as she was having to assist with all the implementation planning while still keeping on top of her normal work. Dr Jones apologised for not realising and offered to get a temp in for a bit to help her out. Kim thanked him for the offer but turned it down as by the time she had explained what needed doing to a temp it would have been quicker to do it herself. Instead she asked for two weeks holiday a few weeks after the system was due to be implemented. Dr Jones agreed to this readily.

Kim agreed to take on the responsibility for backups, managing system maintenance and virus protection and system upgrades.

Installation

The installation of a new system should not have a great effect on the daily running of a practice if it is planned well. Suppliers are used to having to manage the installation with as little imposition on the practice as possible so they will work weekends and out of hours quite readily.

Do make sure that all members of the practice are involved in planning the installation. It only takes one person to have arranged for Mrs Bloggs to come in for an ECG in the middle of the time allocated for installing the hardware in that specific room for all the plans to go askew.

If installation is planned and well prepared for it is possible for most hardware configurations to be set up within a day. Subsequent software set-ups may take a little longer but these can be managed without disrupting the practice.

Avoid staged implementations

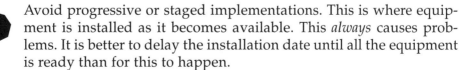

Avoid progressive or staged implementations. This is where equipment is installed as it becomes available. This *always* causes problems. It is better to delay the installation date until all the equipment is ready than for this to happen.

In contrast, it is actually preferable to change staff working patterns in stages as this makes it much easier for them to get used to the new ways of working and their changed role (*see* Chapter 8).

Changing systems and data conversions

It is actually easier to go from a completely paper-based practice to a computerised system than it is for you to change from one system to another. If you are changing from one system to another do be very clear about what will happen to your data.

Generally, suppliers will extract data from your system at an agreed date and time, convert it and load it in your new system ready for when you go live. Subject to your agreeing that you are happy with the conversion this is all well and good – *but*, what happens to patient data in the gap between the extraction and your new system going live? Do find out!

System testing

System testing must be done on your equipment using your data. This sounds obvious but it is amazing how often I hear of practices that have had systems installed and tested using test data or temporary equipment, and it is only after the supplier has left that the problems become apparent. If any bit fails, the whole system has failed. Do not accept anything less than full functionality.

System testing should cover all aspects of your requirements specification even if you are not going to be using parts of it just yet. For example, you may have included a need for pathology links but your local trust is not quite ready for you to connect to them for this. Insist that either this part of your system is tested using an alternative trust or that the supplier will come back and test and finalise the configuration for this when you are ready for it.

If you are a large practice insist on load testing. It is all very well for the system to work with one engineer logged in and with just one set of patient notes being viewed. However, if in practice you are more likely to have up to 20 people logged in at once with over 10 sets of notes being viewed at once, then you need to be sure that the system can cope with this.

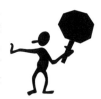

Be pedantic about system testing. It is far easier to get it corrected at this stage than it is for the problem to be identified and fixed at a later date. I can guarantee that if you don't your system will fail at the most inconvenient time possible.

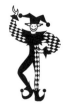

Backup and recovery

System backup and recovery must be tested before the supplier leaves. You should also insist on checking what happens if you have a power failure. It is standard for system servers to be protected by an uninterruptible power suuply (UPS) but this should be tested. Waiting for a real power failure is *not* a valid method of making sure that your server is protected adequately.

New procedures

The new system will almost certainly mean learning new ways of doing things. It is important that these new tasks are agreed and documented. They may include:

- data entry and data checking
- regular system backup and backup testing
- routine system maintenance on servers and workstations
- updating of virus protection software.

Documentation

Everything should be documented clearly. Your new system will come with manuals and guides but do make sure that you write things down for yourself. When you are trying to get to grips with a new system it is far easier to work from your own notes than to rely on official documents.

Encourage staff to make their own notes as well. These will not only be useful for themselves but they will also be a great resource for new staff when they start to get to grips with your system.

Training

There are four types of training that you and your staff should have:

- general computer
- system specific
- coding
- confidentiality.

General computer

General computer training should be provided for anybody who hasn't used a computer before or who is unsure of the new technology. When changing systems it is common to find that staff have never used Windows®-based software before and don't know what to do with the mouse. Your supplier may provide this type of training. If it doesn't ask your PCO ICT manager for help in identifying suitable training, as it will be more than worth the expense. Additionally, some staff may find it useful to attend a short word processing (typing) course.

System specific

Your system supplier will provide some training in the system itself. Generally they will train staff in the parts of the system that they will be using. This is good as far as it goes but means that you have very little skills overlap or redundancy. So if your practice nurse is the only person trained in the chronic disease management templates and protocols and she falls ill, or leaves the practice, anybody taking on her job would not know what to do. Neither would there be anybody who would know enough to show them. Try and ensure that there are always at least two people who know about any part of the system.

Coding

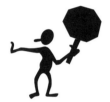

The benefits of an EPR are almost entirely reliant on coding. This means that what ever goes into the system can only be got out again if it is coded. This is great except for the fact that there are often many ways of coding a symptom or disease (*see* Chapter 10, Data recording). Your supplier may provide this type of training. If it doesn't, ask your PCO ICT manager for help in identifying suitable training, as it will be more than worth the expense.

Security and confidentiality

Your system will have a lot of inbuilt security features including the forced use of passwords for all staff. You will need to ensure that all staff are trained in using these facilities but more importantly that they understand why it is so important that they don't share passwords and that they must change them regularly. Once again, your supplier may provide this type of training. If it doesn't, ask your PCO ICT manager for help in identifying suitable training, as any cost is more than outweighed by the potential risks.

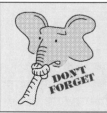

Appendix 10 contains details of a practice-based security policy.

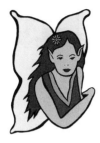 Dr Jones and the rest of the primary care team spent several hours agreeing an implementation plan with their supplier. They were delighted when all their hard work paid off and the installation went very smoothly with little disruption to the practice.

Before the system was installed they all received training on the system itself and in coding and security and confidentiality. Additionally, Dr Andrews and Mandy attended a short course in Windows®, run by the local PCO.

The implementation plan included time for more system-specific training once they had been using the system for a few weeks.

After a few weeks, Mandy and Tracy had the appointments system running smoothly and Tracy was finding that requests for repeat prescriptions could be dealt with very easily and efficiently.

Katy and Alice had run a number of chronic disease clinics and were finding that the use of the computer was making their job much more enjoyable as they didn't have to struggle to remember everything they should check for each patient. Also, if a patient had two conditions they could see the information they had gained from looking at one when looking at the other and no longer did they need to take a patient's blood pressure twice in a week just to check that it was recorded.

Dr Jones took to using the EPR in consultations like a duck to water. Dr Thomas took a few weeks to get to grips with it and more than once could be heard to swear at 'that thing'. Dr Andrews surprised everybody by liking the computer. He was slower than the other doctors and he was still getting to grips with typing.

It was one particular patient that made it all worthwhile for Dr Andrews. A long-standing patient of the practice came in to see him with a sore throat. Dr Andrews had been seeing this patient for this complaint for years and had never been able to convince the patient that there was no need for antibiotics. On this occasion, Dr Andrews duly noted the symptoms and recorded his observations from a physical examination of the patient. He started his normal talk about keeping up the fluids and rest. The patient asked for his prescription. Dr Andrews refused. The normal argument started. Then Dr Andrews remembered the patient advice leaflet on his EPR system and he asked the patient to draw their chair up to the computer. Dr Andrews then called up the leaflet about antibiotic use and showed the patient that '*look, even the computer doesn't think you should have antibiotics*'. The patient stopped arguing, said that '*if the computer says so, it must be right*', and promptly left. Dr Andrews nearly fell off his chair with shock.

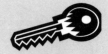

Key points

1 Plan your implementation very carefully.
2 If your chosen supplier does not help you a lot in planning your implementation, think again about your choice of supplier.
3 Think about the healthcare provider, patient, computer screen triangle when planning your physical layouts.
4 Spend time considering how staff roles will change or could change.
5 Data conversions are either very straightforward or hellish!
6 Insist on full system testing – be pedantic!
7 Training, training and more training.

Chapter 7: Future problems you can anticipate

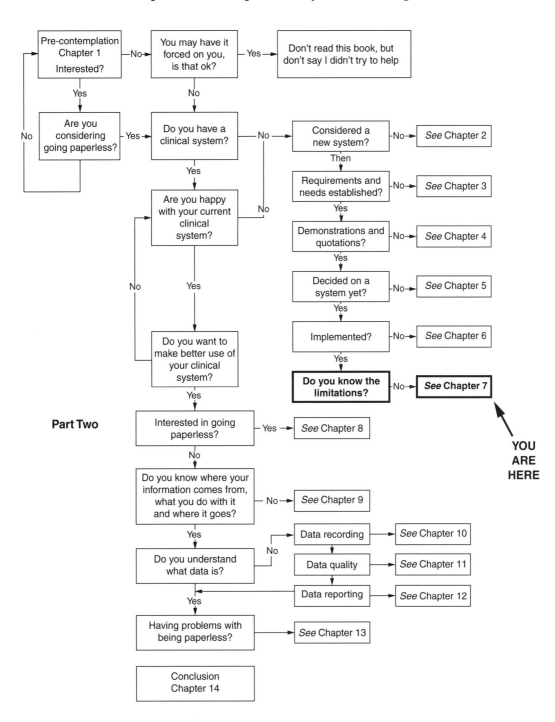

Chapter 7

Future problems you can anticipate

You can't invent events. They just happen. But you have to be prepared to deal with them when they happen.

Constance Baker Motley 1921–

Who should read this chapter?

Either you have just chosen a new computerised EPR system or you are wondering what you forgot to consider when you did.

Training

It is a fact of computerised EPR systems that however much training you have you will always need more. As with other software applications many people never use more than 10% of the capability of an EPR system as they either don't know how to or don't know what is possible. The only way to make really effective use of your system is to consider carefully what you want from it (Part Two) and then to arrange a programme of training for all the practice team that will allow you to meet your needs.

While system-specific training can seem very expensive there are other ways of getting the training you want. First, don't forget your colleagues and friends. If you want to use the system in a specific way, the chances are that they may well have wanted to do the same. In which case, they may have already worked out how to do it.

Second, it may be worth contacting other local practices using the same system to see if they have any staff that need training. You may be able to get the training much cheaper if you can provide a larger group of people to be trained. Alternatively, the system trainer may be able to train on site for you rather than your staff needing to travel to supplier's premises.

Third, and probably most important, are the system user groups. Each of the main suppliers have associated user groups. These are independent of the suppliers but work very closely together. At minimum these national user groups (NUGs) run annual conferences at which you can readily obtain some training. Alternatively, there are usually local user groups (LUGs) that you can join. These usually meet about once a month moving from practice to practice and all sorts of subjects are discussed and looked into.

WWW link	EMIS	http://www.emisnug.org.uk
	IPS	http://www.nvug.org.uk
	Torex Health	http://www.tmug.org.uk

Maintenance

Regular systems maintenance is essential. Your EPR system is like your car. It will keep going if you don't maintain it but over time it will get more and more sluggish and eventually it will just die. Your supplier will train you in carrying out any routine maintenance tasks that need doing. Some of the systems actually run these tasks automatically but you still need to check that they do happen and that they work properly.

Backup

The most important part of regular systems maintenance is daily backup. You *must* make a backup (a copy of your data) at least once a day. That backup, whether on tape or CD ROM should not be stored on site (at the practice) if at all possible. If it must be stored at the practice, make sure it is kept in a fireproof safe. Your supplier will advise you about backup procedures but you should do a backup of any changes at least daily and a full system backup once a week. This means that you should never lose more than a week's data in an absolute worst-case scenario.

Verification and validation
However, it is not enough to simply run a backup. You *must* verify (or validate) that backup regularly. I know of several practices that ran their backups faithfully, even stored the tapes off site (and not on top

of the server thankfully!), but when their system was stolen or broke down and they tried to restore from the backup they found that the tapes were useless as their backup procedure had failed some months previously. If only they had either verified the tapes themselves or arranged for them to be validated by their supplier.

Upgrades

All the suppliers provide regular upgrades to their systems. It is an RFA requirement for the prescribing formulary and Read codes to be upgraded frequently. EMIS will provide these backups automatically over their dial-in or NHSnet 'Patch' system. IPS and Torex currently provide these upgrades on CD ROM. Both have plans for secure remote upgrades in the near future.

However, when you receive these upgrades it is your responsibility to ensure that either they are loaded on your system or to check that they are happening regularly.

Changes in national policy

Unfortunately, as we discussed in Chapter 2, we do not work in isolation. You may have got the best EPR system in the world, be using it as effectively and efficiently as possible, providing excellent and proved patient care and yet you will still have problems.

These may well be beyond your control. Working in the NHS means that we work at the whim of the Government and the powers that be. Should they decide to change national policy, or to change their requirements for primary care computerisation, we will need to adapt and cope with these changes. The best that you can do is to keep half an eye on what is happening nationally and keep in touch with those local to you who are employed to pay specific attention to these things (PCO ICT managers, HA IT managers etc, RHA ICT departments, etc.).

Fortune telling

There are a number of big changes expected in the next few years that will affect primary care computerisation. Some of the most likely are listed below. However, your crystal ball gazing is just as likely to be as accurate as mine.

Read/SNOMED

The first of these is that the Read/SNOMED merger[12] is due to report in late 2001. It is likely that as a result of this all primary care EPR systems will have to convert their systems to SNOMED clinical terms rather than Read version 1 or 2.

It is intended that all existing Read codes will be included in the SNOMED clinical terms and that all your existing data will be readily converted. However, the clinical terms do not use the hierarchical structures of Read version 1 and 2 and you will either need to learn new methods of coding or the suppliers will need to make coding much less transparent in their systems.

GP to GP transfer

There are a number of projects working on the problem of electronically transferring patient records between practices. It is likely that a solution will be agreed in the next few years and that suppliers will need to upgrade their systems to account for this.

Electronic prescribing

As with GP to GP transfer there are a number of projects working out the problems inherent in electronic prescribing. It is likely that one of these will result in an agreed solution within the next few years. Again, suppliers will need to upgrade their systems to account for this.

Electronic health record (EHR)

At some point, a decision will be made about the EHR and whether it is a synthesis of multiple EPRs or not, and how it is created and who maintains and owns it. When these decisions are made, they will have implications for primary care. It is hoped that as primary care has far more experience of clinical computing than other health domains, the lessons learned there will not need to be repeated. Hopefully, this will mean that the consequences for primary care will be reduced.

Remember that you are paying your supplier to sort out these problems. However, you will have new training needs to deal with.

Key points

1 You can never have enough training.
2 Maintain your system.
3 Backup daily.
4 Validate your backups and store them safely.
5 Make sure that your system is upgraded regularly.
6 Practice crystal ball gazing.

Part Two

Going paperless

Chapter 8: Going paperless

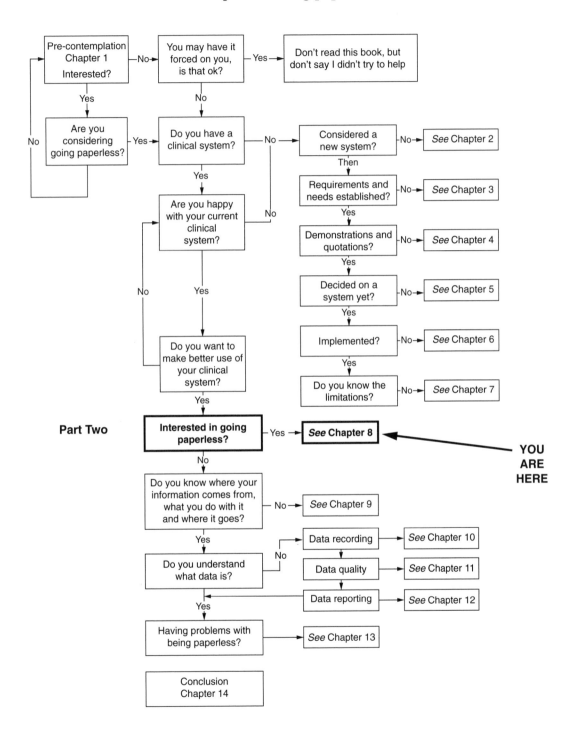

Going paperless

If you really want to reach for the brass ring, just remember that there are sacrifices that go along.

Cathleen Blake

Who should read this chapter?

You should read this chapter if you are interested in going paperless but are unsure as to what it actually means.

What does 'paperless practice' mean?

A paperless practice is one that records all medical records and prescribing on an EPR. They do *not* use Lloyd George notes for anything other than storing historical medical records and copies of paper letters and reports from other organisations. All referrals and test results are recorded or generated from within the EPR.

The usual reason for wanting to go paperless is that you have spent thousands of pounds on an EPR system and you want to get all the benefits you were promised from it. In which case, you are in one of three groups.

1 You have either just purchased an EPR system for the first time or you have recently changed your EPR system (hopefully, you have done this with the support of Part One of this book).
2 You have had an EPR system for some time but don't think that you are making the best use of it.
3 You have been held back from going paperless before but now have an opportunity to do it properly.

The ABC Health Centre has had their new EPR system in place now for about three months. The reception staff are still delighted at how much easier it is to manage appointments and requests for repeat prescriptions. The patients seem to have been quite happy with the new system and all the doctors are now running full clinics again (they had reduced the number of patients they could see for the first few weeks after implementation to give themselves time to get used to using the system in consultation).

However, the clinical staff have found that they can't always find the information they want on the computer system.

At the primary care team meeting Dr Jones asked everybody what they thought of the new system. Katy and Alice (nurse practitioner and practice nurse) said that they didn't think they were using it as effectively as they could be. Dr Thomas commented that it didn't seem to be as easy to enter data as it looked when the system was demonstrated.

Dr Jones suggested that this was probably because the demo system had been set up to make data entry easy with lots of short cut keys and templates.

Dr Jones suggested that they visit a local beacon practice that was using the same EPR system as them. They all thought that this would be a great idea and Dr Jones arranged for them all to spend an afternoon with the Beacon site.

The Beacon site they visited was a paperless practice. At the next primary care team meeting all the ABC Health Centre staff were really enthusiastic about 'going paperless' too. They agreed that they would work towards becoming paperless within the next six months.

Dr Andrews was concerned about the legal status of a full EPR. Dr Jones reminded him that they had checked this out when they were looking at getting a new clinical system. They had received approval from their HA to keep some of their records electronically. Dr Jones would now write to the HA again and ask for approval to move towards keeping all of their records on the computer.

Legal status

From a medico-legal position a paperless practice is actually better than a paper-based one. All systems accredited to RFA99[6] must have an inbuilt audit trail. This audit trail records everything that happens within the clinical system. So if you log in to your system and look at patient A's notes, review patient B's medication and then issue a repeat prescription for patient C, this is all recorded. Your identity (provided by your logging in) is logged, as is what you did and the time and date of your activity.

Hopefully, you will never need to use the audit trail and for added security it is not usually accessible to anybody but system suppliers experts. You may be interested to know that the legal status of the audit trail was recognised in court during the Shipman case.[13]

The major barrier to becoming paperless used to be the GP terms of service requirement for paper-based records. However, this was amended in October 2000 and all GPs can now maintain all or part of their record on a computer system as long as they have the approval of their HA.[14]

Data Protection Act

All PCOs, including general practices, must register with the data protection commissioner. Ask your PCO for help with your registration and remember that you must not only obey the act but also keep your registration up to date.

WWW link   http://www.dataprotection.gov.uk/

Do not destroy paper files

Just one word of caution, some paperless practices either scan or enter details from incoming letters and then destroy the paper originals. We shall look at where all the information comes from and what to do with it later on. However, do *not* destroy your paper copies as all UK medical defence unions currently advocate keeping them on file. Hopefully, it won't be long before all this information is being transmitted electronically and the letters will cease to exist on paper.

Preparation for going paperless

Before you can go paperless there are a number of ground rules that you need to agree. The following list of ground rules is based on those developed by the PRIM-IS project.[15]

Five ground rules to consider before going paperless

1 *Remember the purpose*
The primary purpose of recording information is to support patient care. If the information you agree to record is not required routinely for patient care, it is unlikely to be recorded consistently or completely, particularly in the longer term.

2 *All members of the primary care team must take part in data recording*
If just one member of the team does not participate in data recording you will not be recording information about the full practice population. If you don't do this, clinical audit, practice planning and commissioning is very difficult and it is impossible to calculate rates of incidence and prevalence of disease.

GPs and other clinicians *must* enter their own data directly onto the computer system, as this reduces problems of transcription error and legibility.

3 *All contact with patients must be recorded*
To obtain a full picture of practice morbidity, you must record data gained from locums, trainees, phone calls and from encounters outside the consulting room, such as home visits.

4 *Consistent recording*
Each episode of illness should be coded with only one code, to avoid multiple diagnoses being counted. This means that clinicians should not record asthma in one instance and asthmatic bronchitis in another, unless the diagnosis has actually changed.

5 *Regular feedback and audit*
Unless data quality is regularly audited and the findings of the audits acted upon, the data will lack credibility in analyses. Audits on a quarterly basis are recommended for at least the first two years after a practice decides to go paperless. We will look at methods that can be used to audit data quality later on.

Source: Section 3.2 *Standards in Collection of Health Data from General Practice (CHDGP) Guidelines* (2000). NHS IA, Exeter. http://www.nottingham.ac.uk/chdgp/

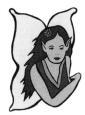 Dr Jones discussed the five ground rules with the primary care team. They agreed that only recording information they needed for patient care was an important principle and all the staff repeated their commitment to all using the EPR system. However, they realised that they hadn't been thinking about the information that was being lost on home visits, phone calls and when they had locum cover.

They were still not really sure of this coding lark or how they could actually look at their data quality. Kim mentioned that she had seen something about a national project that was looking at these things. She thought it was called PRIMIS and offered to find out more about it to see if it would be any use to them.

They agreed that at the next meeting they would draw up a plan for going paperless. Dr Jones said that he would ask the PCO ICT manager if she could attend this meeting to help them with this. The PCO ICT manager was delighted to be asked and suggested that she bring a copy of a plan that she had used before for them to look at.

Planning for going paperless

Just like when you were thinking about getting, or changing, your EPR system and you needed to spend a lot of time in planning and thinking about it before you actually bought a system, you need to spend a lot of time thinking and planning before going paperless. It is much easier to start with recording a little bit of information well and increase the amount you record over time than it is to put it right if you record a lot of information in a poor way.

Just a thought! Do remember that Dr Jones' practice is a fairy story. It is likely that it will take you *much* longer than six months to go paperless. The average seems to be about two to three years and I know a practice that swears that it takes ten years to do it properly!

I think the 26 weeks plan detailed in Appendix 11 is very optimistic. However, it does break the tasks down very nicely and will give you a good idea of the things you need to consider.

The PCO ICT manager sent Dr Jones a copy of the plan she had mentioned for going paperless. She explained that it had been designed to help GPs and nurses who were not using their practice computer during consultations. She realised that the ABC Health Centre was quite a long way through this plan but thought they might find it interesting to look at. Dr Jones thought it might help to identify areas they needed to think more about.

Appendix 11 contains a copy of a 26-week plan for going paperless developed by Kathie Applebee.[16]

Key points

1 Going paperless means that you will record *everything* in your EPR. You will not use Lloyd George notes for anything but historical reference and for filing paper copies of documentation received by the practice.
2 You must have the approval of your HA to go paperless.
3 You must register under the Data Protection Act and keep to its requirements.
4 Do not destroy paper copies of documentation received by the practice.
5 There are five ground rules to consider when preparing to go paperless.
6 Develop a plan to go paperless. If you try to do everything in one go you will find it virtually impossible.

Chapter 9: Information sources, uses and destinations

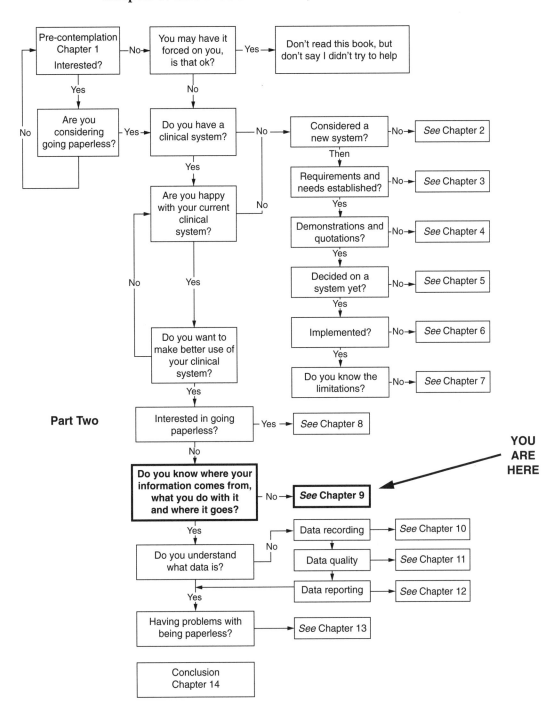

Information sources, uses and destinations

It is a capital mistake to theorise before one has data.
Scandal in Bohemia
Sir Arthur Conan Doyle 1859–1930

Who should read this chapter?

You either have a new EPR system or have realised that you are not using your old one very effectively. In order to make the most of your EPR you need to identify where all your information comes from, what you do with it and where it goes.

Where does your information come from?

Before you can decide how you are going to deal with information electronically in your practice, you need to identify where it comes from. You will probably assume that the vast majority of it will come from your primary care team. However, this is not always the case and you will need to consider how you deal with information from other sources.

Primary care team

A primary care team generally has far more members than just the GP partners. If you think about it, I think you'll find that all your staff are involved in collecting and recording data about patients.

This means that you need to think about what this means for your data for all of the following people:

- GP partners
- locums
- GP registrars (formerly known as GP trainees)
- practice nurses
- nurse practitioners
- community nurses
- health visitors
- counsellors
- peripatetic specialist nurses, e.g. diabetes liaison nurses
- community psychiatric nurses
- practice management
- reception staff
- clerical staff.

This above list is almost certainly not complete as you may have other staff using your EPR.

You might decide that some of the people listed don't have any serious input into the collection of data in your practice. If this is the case, why don't you think about why this is? Is it because they don't need to, they don't want to or they can't with the way the system is set up at the moment?

It is often the case that community staff would love to use the GP EPR systems at the practices they work with but either they don't have the skills or they aren't given the opportunity. Is this the case for your practice? Are you happy with this?

Within the primary care team you will need to consider how to record information gained from the following:

- members of the PCT, who do not routinely use the system
- locum staff who are unfamiliar with the practice computer system
- home visits, out-of-hours consultations and consultations at branch surgeries
- if the computer system goes down
- information generated by other organisations (e.g. test results, hospital admissions).

Clinical staff must check cleric data entry

One of the ways many practices deal with these sort of issues is to use clerical staff to record information from written notes placed in input baskets or boxes. However, the accuracy of patient data on the system is a clinical responsibility. If you choose to do this, clinicians *must* check both the accuracy of data entered by clerical staff and *clinicians* must check that agreed procedures are being stuck to.

Data coming from outside the practice

Not all your data comes from your primary care team. There is a lot of information that comes into your practice from outside. This can come from all sorts of places such as:

- out-of-hours service – information can come from people dealing with your patients on your behalf such as a deputising service, an informal arrangement with another practice or an out-of-hours co-operative
- laboratory reports
- clinical letters, e.g. outpatient attendances, admissions, laboratory results, hospital discharge letters, etc.
- clinical data on patients who transfer onto the practice list from another practice
- reports from accident and emergency departments
- patients – patients may well write, email, call or fax you with information that you need to record without actually seeing the patient
- interventions carried out elsewhere.

Information sources

Write a list of all the places and types of people that you get information from. You can then use this to decide what you want to record and how it will be recorded.

At the primary care team meeting everybody had a look at the 26-week plan. They decided that they were actually just over half way down this plan, although they hadn't been that systematic at using their EPR system. All prescribing was being done on the EPR and they did try and record the reason for the consultation and the results of any examinations. Where they had got stuck was on using things like templates and different screens.

The PCO ICT manager then asked them to list all the places and people that they get information from. This was quite quick and easy although the list was a lot longer than they had thought it would be.

The PCO ICT manager then suggested that they think about what information they *needed* to know from all these sources.

What do you do with your information?

You now have an idea of where all your information comes from but do you know what you do with it?

Have a look at your list of information sources and see if you can identify for each one what happens to it. You must do this with the full primary care team otherwise you will find that there will be some piece of information that just one person in the team deals with and it will get missed out.

Where does your information go?

You now have a list of where all your information comes from and an idea of what happens to it within your practice but what about information that you give to other people?

If you think about it for a moment, you are constantly giving information to other people and places. Every time you refer a patient or a patient moves away from your practice you give away information.

Generally, you will also have to give information to your PCO or HA. If nothing else, you will have to provide some form of annual report that will include information on your patient population and chronic disease. It is likely that you are also giving information to some form of data collection or data quality project (e.g. PRIMIS).

How do you manage your chronic disease registers? Do you keep them on your own system or do you give information to some central point?

Take another look at your list of information and now that you have worked out what you do with it also think about where you send it.

You should end up being able to list for every possible type of information that your primary care team deals with.

- Where does it come from?
- What do you do with it?
- Where does it go?

Chronic disease registers

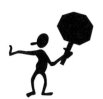

A note of caution. There is a great deal of pressure on primary care to create and maintain chronic disease registers as part of the NSF requirements. There is no need for you to send this information to a central database to do this. If you are using your EPR system fully, your register is automatically created within your system. All you need to do is to run a search or report.[17]

If you must send information outside of the practice for this type of work you *must* have explicit informed consent from each patient. Personally, I would also insist that this information was always anonymised. Likewise, any data collection or data quality project does not need identifiable information and you should only provide anonymised information if you take part in any of these schemes.

Of course, you do need to provide identifiable information for referrals or pathology requests. However, do think about the information you provide and check that you are conforming to your own Data Protection Act registration.

The primary care team looked at their list of all the places they got information from. They then took each one in turn and everybody in the team listed what they did with that information. The doctors were quite surprised at how much of the information the nurses used. They then listed all the different places and people that they sent information to.

There were a few things that they decided they were not happy about and decided that they would change the way they had been working. Kim (practice manager) wrote up all of their lists and decisions so that they could use it to develop data recording guidelines.

Key points

1 Your primary care team is bigger than you think. List all the members.
2 List all the places and people that you get information from (both from outside the practice and from your primary care team).
3 Work out what you currently do with all this information.
4 List all the places and people that you send information to.
5 If in doubt, do not send or give patient-identifiable data to anybody.
6 Remember that you must have informed consent from each patient for their details to be given to somebody else, even if that is only for the HA to maintain a disease register.

Chapter 10: Data recording

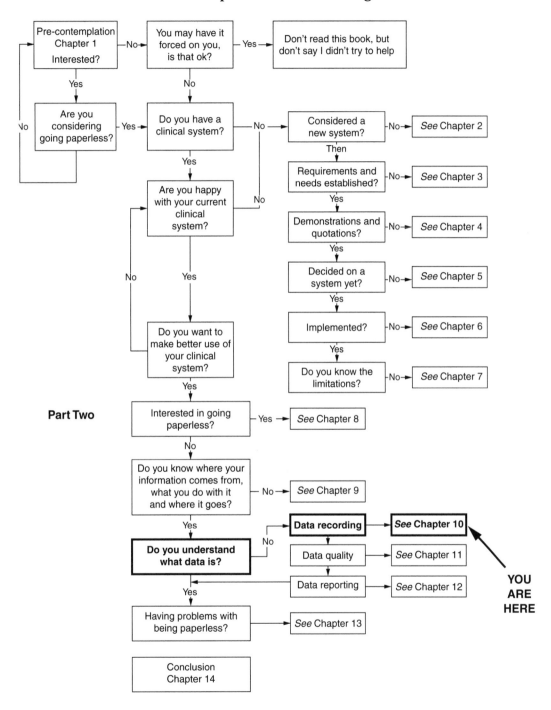

Pre-contemplation
Chapter 1
Interested?

—No→

You may have it
forced on you,
is that ok?

—Yes→

Don't read this book, but
don't say I didn't try to help

Yes ↓   No ↓

Are you
considering
going paperless?

—Yes→

Do you have a
clinical system?

—No→

Considered a
new system?

—No→ *See* Chapter 2

Then

Requirements and
needs established?

—No→ *See* Chapter 3

No ↓

Are you happy
with your current
clinical
system?

No→

Yes

Demonstrations and
quotations?

—No→ *See* Chapter 4

Yes

Decided on a
system yet?

—No→ *See* Chapter 5

Yes

Do you want to
make better use of
your clinical
system?

Implemented?

—No→ *See* Chapter 6

Yes

Do you know the
limitations?

—No→ *See* Chapter 7

Yes ↓

Part Two

Interested in going
paperless?

— Yes → *See* Chapter 8

No ↓

Do you know where your
information comes from,
what you do with it
and where it goes?

— No → *See* Chapter 9

Yes ↓

Data recording → *See* **Chapter 10**

No

**Do you understand
what data is?**

Data quality → *See* Chapter 11

Data reporting → *See* Chapter 12

**YOU
ARE
HERE**

Yes ↓

Having problems with
being paperless?

→ *See* Chapter 13

Conclusion
Chapter 14

Data recording

I never lose an opportunity of urging a practical start, however small, for it is wonderful how often the mustard seed germinates and roots itself.

Florence Nightingale 1820–1910

Who should read this chapter?

You have decided to go paperless and you want to develop procedures to make sure you record all the information you need. You have identified all the places and people that give you information and now you need to decide how you are going to deal with all that data.

What are you doing now?

Before you can decide how you are going to deal with the data, you need to find out what you are doing now. It is likely, unless you have thought about this before, that everybody has developed their own view on what should be recorded, how it is recorded and who records it when.

You need to answer the following questions.

- What information is recorded by the practice?
- How is it recorded?
- Who records it?
- When do they record it?
- What isn't being recorded at the moment that you need?
- What are your current recording policies, if any?

Appendix 3 gives you details of GPIMM, which is a tool that will help you look at what you do with your data now.

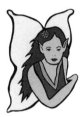

When the primary care team started to think about what information they needed to know from all the people and places that gave them data they realised that they didn't know what was being recorded now. They decided to go through their list and make a note of what was recorded from the information coming in to the practice. They then made a list of all the things they felt were important to know. From this they could identify all the information that was just getting lost at the moment and all the inconsistencies in how they dealt with the information.

They found that while all the doctors were now using the computer in their consultations, only Dr Jones was recording all the things that they all thought should be recorded. Dr Andrews was really only recording prescriptions and major morbidities. Likewise, while the nurses had taken on chronic disease management they discovered that Katy was recording things differently from Alice.

What to record?

Going paperless means that you have decided to rely on your EPR as your *only* source of patient information. Therefore, when you are thinking about what to record your first thought should be *What do I need to know to support patient care?*

However, there are a few other things that will effect your decision about what you need to record. For example, some of the NSFs require practices to maintain chronic disease registers. These often include minimum datasets. You may decide to record something specifically to be able to audit it within your practice. You may also need to record something just to help you understand the needs of your practice population.

To get you started in thinking about what you need to record, have a look at the two lists below:

Contact information

For each contact with a patient you should record at least the following.

- *Date of consultation*: this is usually generated automatically by the system. However you should be careful to check that the default is not used inappropriately, e.g. for a home visit entered later.

- *Author*: this is usually generated automatically by the system and based on the identifier used to log in to the system. This is used for queries and audit but more importantly forms part of the audit trail.
- *Morbidity or problem*: these should be Read coded.
- *Risk factors*: these should be Read coded.
- *Examination results*: such as blood pressure, PFR, etc.

Patient information

For each patient you need to think about how you will record the following.

- *Patient demographics*: date of birth, sex, postcode, ID of registered GP, patient ID, date of registration, date of leaving, HA area the patient lives in.
- *Morbidities*: must be consistently Read coded.
- *Lifestyle and risk factors*.
- *Medication*: acute or repeat, date of prescription, drug code, quantity prescribed, route, cost, ID of prescribing GP.
- *Referrals*: ID of referring GP, date of referral, diagnosis or symptom (Read coded), referral type, provider ID, reason for referral.
- *Interventions carried out outside practice*: date of hospital event, author, confirmed diagnosis, results of investigations, tests, procedures, location, medication.
- *Outpatient letters, discharge summaries, results*.

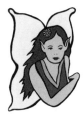

The primary care team decided that they needed recording guidelines for the practice. They listed all the things that they agreed should be recorded, where it came from and who should record it. They also agreed that wherever possible the clinicians would record the data during consultations. The doctors also agreed to enter anything they wanted in the record that came from external documents.

They were fortunate in that their new system used pathology links and all their path results were dealt with automatically by the system.

They agreed that they would start using the system to generate referral letters. Alice and Katy decided to find out more about templates and protocols so that they could be sure that they were recording consistently.

It soon became apparent during these discussions that nobody really understood Read codes. Kim (practice manager) offered to arrange for training for all the staff in Read coding. This was thought to be an excellent idea and soon arranged.

Coding

Since the late 1980s all GP EPR systems have used clinical coding to store information. All this means is that when you want to enter a medical term or a concept (e.g. blood pressure, asthma, etc.) the EPR system will offer you a set of 'terms' or 'rubrics', together with 'codes'. You can then choose from this list and the information is recorded.

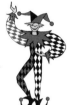

The advantage of codes is that the computer can understand them, which means that you can search and find anything you want to know about your patients – as long as you have recorded it of course! If you don't use codes (free text) you can **not** get this information back out of your system.

RFA accredited systems use Read codes for all aspects of clinical work. However you will find that some systems will use other coding systems for recording medication and appliances. Generally these will be coded using either the BNF codes (*British National Formulary*) or system-specific codes, for example the EMIS drug codes.

Although Read codes are now the NHS standard for primary care you will soon find that you can code many things in a variety of ways. This tends to undermine the value of coding and the only way of dealing with it is to agree coding protocols. You might agree this for your own practice or you could make use of established codes. For example, the PRIMIS project (*see* Chapter 11, Data quality) provides a list of recommended codes for core morbidities that you could use. Additionally, there are now datasets being produced nationally for each of the NSFs. You can find these in the condition-specific information strategies that are associated with each NSF.

The more you can learn about coding the better. Ideally, you would never need to see the actual codes and it would all happen behind the scenes. However, this isn't the way current systems work unless you make use of templates and protocols.

Appendix 12 gives you a brief guide to the Read codes and some examples you can work through to get to know them better.

SNOMED/Read merger

Just to make sure you are kept on your toes the NHS is currently working with an American coding system, SNOMED, with the intention that the new coding system, which is a combination of Read and SNOMED, called SNOMED CT (clinical terms) will be completed by the end of 2001 and implemented across the NHS.[12]

We have been assured that SNOMED CT will be completely compatible with existing versions of Read.

The main problem with this will be a big headache for your system supplier, as they will need to do a lot of work on their system to move to SNOMED CT. For now, learn all you can about Read and coding and just watch to see what happens.

WWW link   http://www.doh.gov.uk/

Recording guidelines

Once you have decided what you need to record, the primary care team should develop practice recording guidelines, which are agreed and accepted by all members. These guidelines should be comprehensive and directed towards the practice's target recording level. Your guidelines should make sure that appropriate codes are being used.

The guidelines should include the following.

- What is to be recorded?
- When is it to be recorded?
- Who is it to record it?
- How is it to be recorded?
- What codes should be used?

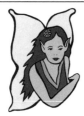

Kim (practice manager) arranged for all the members of the primary care team to attend training on Read coding.

At the next primary care team meeting they agreed that they needed a list of 'best codes' for the things they recorded most often. Mandy knew that one of her friends worked in a practice that was taking part in the PRIMIS project and said she would see if she could have a copy of their list of codes.

The primary care team looked through these codes at the next team meeting. The doctors were unhappy with one or two of the suggestions and felt that they would like more detail. They looked up alternative codes on their EPR.

Kim typed up the revised list and a copy was placed by every screen so that everybody could use the same codes.

When to record?

It is important that you think about all the possible ways in which you have contact with your patients. Every contact is a possible source of information that you may need to know. If you don't consider all possibilities you may well miss recording important information.

You have opportunities to gain information about a patient when they:

- register with the practice
- have a routine health check: cervical smear, blood pressure check, etc.
- consult you for a perceived health problem
- consult you for a recurring problem
- are pregnant
- consult you for a service, such as immunisation or contraception
- consult you for advice
- visit them at home.

 You can either record directly or indirectly. I strongly recommend direct data entry as it reduces errors and involves the clinician entering information about a patient at the time of the consultation. However, be warned – direct data entry can be very time-consuming until you become familiar with the way your system works.

Direct data entry – in consultation

When recording during consultations, the following PRIMIS 'tips' may be helpful:[18]

PRIMIS 'tips'

- Phase in use of Read codes, perhaps recording only significant morbidities first and moving on to record all morbidities and symptoms over time.
- Lists of Read codes for common conditions can be very helpful, both in terms of speeding consultation and ensuring consistency. They may be kept on paper beside the computer or, where the facility is available on the practice system, incorporated into picking lists.
- Use templates or protocols if your system supports them.
- If an appropriate Read code or term cannot be found during the consultation, put the notes to one side for coding after surgery.
- Make full use of synonyms to make code selection easier, e.g. OM for acute otitis media. Some systems allow users to set up their own synonyms; caution is recommended to practices wishing to do this, to ensure that local synonyms are appropriately linked and fully understood by all users.

- Try to be consistent in the Read code used for the same condition.
- Identify an individual in the practice who is the most proficient at and interested in using Read codes to become an adviser for the rest of the practice.

Source: Section 5.3 *Collection of Health Data from General Practice (CHDGP) Guidelines* (2000). NHS IA, Exeter. http://www.nottingham.ac.uk/chdgp/

Indirect data entry

Data entry by clinicians at the point of care is recommended wherever possible. However, unless you have some form of mobile computing (e.g. a laptop or hand-held that can hold either a full copy of your patient database or at least parts of it) you will need to think about how you want to deal with home visits. You also need to decide how you are going to deal with all that other information gained from outside the practice.

Generally practices deal with these issues by developing procedures that involve the data being entered onto the practice computer system by clerical staff. I really don't recommend this but if you *must* use clerical staff then it is very important that your clerical staff have adequate training and support in both your clinical system and coding. In particular, you must identify a clinician that they can ask about coding issues and be explicit about what documents should be routed to whom and what should be recorded.

Practices using indirect data entry often find that their data quality is very poor due to legibility and transcription errors. The following PRIMIS 'tips' may help reduce these problems:[19]

PRIMIS 'tips'

- Check back in the notes to make sure that the same name is used for a condition that has been recorded previously.
- Use templates or protocols to assist data entry.
- Provide a list of Read codes, where the clinician can simply record the appropriate code or term.
- Use the diagnosis symbol (D) or highlight problems to identify within the notes relevant information for recording.
- Write the details to be recorded on a separate form, such as an appointment list, with space to add problems.
- Dictate problems during or after consultation.
- Have different coloured boxes to indicate which notes have yet to be routed through the input clerk prior to re-filing.

- Once data has been entered, a highlighter pen or red tick can be used to identify it as having been entered. This procedure acts as a check on the system and will assist scanning of the notes during a consultation.
- Where a diagnosis needs to be changed, the patient's notes must be clearly amended.
- To identify that data has been entered on behalf of a clinician by clerical staff, the identifier used to log in to the system should be set up to identify the clerk concerned. The clinician should be identified separately in the consultation details.
- Setting data capture targets along the lines of 'all information placed in the box for data entry by the end of the day will be entered into the system by the end of the next day' is strongly recommended to avoid backlogs developing.
- Identify a coding adviser for the rest of the practice.

Source: Section 5.4 *Collection of Health Data from General Practice (CHDGP) Guidelines* (2000). NHS IA, Exeter. http://www.nottingham.ac.uk/chdgp/

System failures

There is one other situation that I didn't mention before where you will need to rely on indirect data entry. That is if your system fails catastrophically. Ideally, this will never happen and if it does, you will have followed the guidance for backup and maintenance and you will be up and running again very quickly. However, you should have contingency plans in the event of a prolonged system failure or power cut. These should include alternative data recording methods. For example, data collection forms could be used, with agreed places to store completed forms and staff identified to enter the data once the system is running again.

Consistency

All staff must agree on the method you will use for data entry. It might be possible to allow some members of the team to use one method and some the other, but any decision to allow indirect data entry must be clear about what is to be entered and by whom. Where both direct and indirect data entry is happening within the same practice, it is important that all members of the practice are applying the same rules.

Any disagreements between clinicians about data entry, coding or commitment to going paperless must be identified, faced and reconciled.

How to record?

If you have decided to go paperless you have by default decided to record electronically all data, from whatever source, that you have agreed that you *need* to record.

The best procedures for entering information that has come from outside the practice is for a GP to read the letter or report and to enter the information on the patient's EPR themselves. However, if the GP really can't do this an alternative method is for the GP to highlight the parts of the letter or report that need to be entered in the EPR. Clerical staff can then code and enter this information as long as they have suitable support and advice on coding. The GP will still be responsible for this information and will need to personally assure themselves as to the accuracy and consistency of their clerical staff.

Use of templates and protocols

All the major GP EPR systems include templates or protocols. However, the systems do vary in what they call them and how they work. For example:

- some of the systems allow templates or protocols to be 'linked' to a particular Read code, so that when that code is entered, an appropriate template or protocol is displayed as a reminder of the information required
- some systems provide standard templates and protocols
- some systems allow you to develop your own templates and protocols designed to suit the clinical guidelines of your practice.

Well-constructed templates and protocols are a valuable aid for clinical care. You should find out what templates or protocols for the core morbidities and risk factors are on your clinical system. If they are available, you should check that they use the codes you want to use. You may find that protocols are called something else by some of the suppliers. For example, they are called SOPHIEs in Torex System 6000 and Clinical Decision Support in In Practice System's Vision.

Templates

A template is a data entry screen, which prompts you to record certain items in certain clinical situations. For example, an asthma template may prompt you to enter symptoms and triggers for the patient. As well as providing a prompt for the information, a template should also enter the agreed code into the patient's record. A template is like a computerised paper data entry form.

Templates can be used:

- to make data entry much faster
- to ensure that all appropriate information about a patient is obtained

- to check that information is recorded consistently across the practice.

Templates can also provide 'picking lists' of appropriate Read terms to simplify selection. Templates are most often used to support monitoring of patients with chronic diseases and in other clinic and health promotion sessions. For example, a template for diabetes might include data capture on risk factors, interventions, management methods, medication and complications, to provide a complete picture of patient care, including outcomes.

Protocols

A protocol is very similar, but it allows you to do a few extra things:

- it lets you skip items automatically when they are not appropriate (e.g. not asking a non-smoker how many cigarettes they smoke)
- it will offer different options depending on the data you have entered (e.g. if a patient smokes and is overweight, the protocol might suggest taking a cholesterol test)
- it can provide a printout of advice to the patient, tailored to their condition.

Decision support

Before we leave the subject of protocols we should look at decision support very briefly. There are many definitions of decision support and how it can be implemented in GP clinical systems. For example, some of the things that are considered as decision support are:

- systems that use prompts that alert you to data that requires collection
- systems that use templates to require specific information, usually used in disease clinics
- systems that offer online access to electronic formularies, textbooks, differential diagnosis software, printing patient advice leaflets.

PRODIGY

Whether you think these are clinical decision support systems or not, one issue that is more controversial is the use of online treatment protocols. These appear during the consultation usually in response to a trigger and before the clinician initiates management. Their approach is based on the principle that effective treatment is evidence-based and relies on the assumption that the information provided is up to date. The most obvious example of an online treatment protocol is the one mandated within RFA99, PRODIGY. All RFA99 accredited systems have the ability to offer PRODIGY to its users. Some doctors feel that PRODIGY reduces autonomy; others feel that it aids, rather than replaces, the decision-making process.

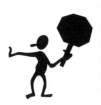

WWW link   http://www.prodigy.nhs.uk/

Scanning

Some paperless practices scan all documents that come into the practice that contain patient information. They then attach these scanned documents to the patient's EPR. *This is a waste of time!* At the moment you can not search or retrieve patient information from these scanned images electronically. This means that if you want to be paperless and make full use of your system, you still need to manually code and enter on the EPR the information you need from these documents. Scanning the document simply means that you will be duplicating your workload and consuming large amounts of storage space on your hard drive. This isn't even offset by the possibility of destroying the original paper documents as medico-legally the medical defence unions still advise you to retain them.

Katy and Alice (nurse practitioner and practice nurse) were concerned that they weren't recording the same things or in the same way. One of Alice's friends had mentioned that she used a lot of templates.

Katy and Alice arranged to go and see Alice's friend who showed them the templates she used. She had started with the ones provided with her system and then edited them to make them more suitable for how she liked to work. Katy and Alice thought these were great and had a look at the templates on their own system. Within a few hours they had agreed which ones they wanted to use and had made some minor changes to check that the templates would automatically put the codes the practice wanted to use in the record.

Key points

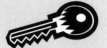

1 Look at your current recording policies, if any.
2 Identify what you *need* to know, and thus what you must record.
3 Learn how to code.
4 Decide on your preferred method of data entry – direct or indirect.
5 Decide how you are going to treat data coming from outside the practice.
6 Develop practice policies for data recording – consistency is the key.
7 Find out what templates or protocols are available for you to use, and make more use of them. Edit them if necessary!
8 Reconcile any significant disagreements between clinicians concerning data recording.
9 Do not scan documents.

Chapter 11: Data quality

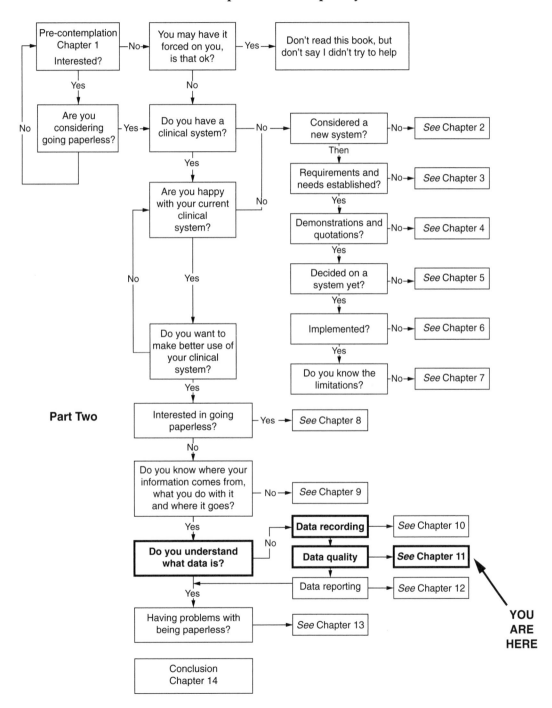

Data quality

Yard by yard it's very hard. But inch by inch, it's a cinch.

Anon

Who should read this chapter?

Anybody who is using a computerised system for recording any part of their patients' notes should be interested in finding out about the quality of the information they are recording. Once you know what quality it is you can then work on making it better.

What is data quality?

PRIMIS, the national project concerned primarily with the quality of computerised data in primary care describes good quality data as:

*   accurate
*   complete
*   relevant
*   up to date
*   accessible.

One of the biggest problems in going paperless is making sure that your information is complete. By complete, I mean that all members of your PCT always record everything you have agreed needs to be recorded for every patient. In reality, you are likely to find that some people record some information, about some patients, on some days of the week.

How can I be sure that my data is good quality?

There are a number of things you can do to be sure that your data is good quality. The most important of these you have already started by developing data recording guidelines. By following these you are making sure that you are recording accurately and consistently.

The next thing you can do is look at the data already on your system. It is likely that your data is not complete or accurate, either because you haven't been using it for very long and haven't got a lot of information on the system yet or because you have a lot of information on the system but have never considered the quality of it before.

If you are in the first group you may not need to do much work to check the quality of your data. If you are in the second, I am afraid you may need to spend a lot of time checking your data.

The best way of checking your data is to review each patient's notes. However, this is the real world and it is very unlikely that you will have the time do this. Fortunately there are a few other things you can do.

Dr Jones was concerned that his partners had mentioned being unable to find some things when they wanted to. He was very pleased that the primary care team had agreed data recording guidelines but decided that he wanted to check the quality of the data already on their system.

He made a list of a few things that he wanted to check, such as males with hysterectomies or females with testicular disease. He also wanted to look at specific medications.

With Kim's (practice manager) help, he ran a number of searches that identified different groups of patients that didn't seem quite right. He then reviewed each of their notes himself. If necessary, he asked Tracy and Mandy (receptionists) to pull the paper notes so that he could check what should be on the system.

Fortunately, as they hadn't been using the system that long and they had only had their patient demographics, prescribing and register data imported from their old system, there was very little that needed to be put right. Within a few days Dr Jones was happy that whilst they had very little information on the system what they had was now OK. With their new recording guidelines he was sure that as the information was added it would be of good quality too. However, he asked Kim to re-run the searches they had written in six months time just to check.

Dr Jones was still a little concerned about his partner's comments and asked Dr Andrews to explain what he had meant. When Dr Andrews showed Dr Jones what he meant it was soon easy to see that it was simply because of the way the screen was laid out. Dr Jones showed Dr Andrews and Dr Thomas how they could choose which parts of the records they could see when they were looking at a patient's notes.

You can run regular reviews of your data. Like Dr Jones and Kim, once you have set up searches that look for odd things and things that just don't make sense you can simply re-run them every few months. The sort of things you can look for are as follows.

- The wrong codes being used. You can search for codes that have been entered that should not have been used. This is useful when you are trying to make sure that you all use the same codes.
- No diagnostic code but indicator present. For example, you may like to search for all patients with high or raised blood pressure codes but who do not have a diagnostic code for hypertension.
- Overdue recall dates. Patients may not have been for a consultation or the flag may not have been removed.
- Indicators not recorded in a specified time period. For example, diagnosed hypertensives that have not had their blood pressure recorded in the last 12 months.
- Compare your data with your PACT data. This can only provide a very crude check, i.e. if the amount of a particular drug dispensed is higher than that prescribed, medication is not being completely recorded on the system.
- The number of consultations that do not have a problem recorded.
- Patients with morbidity incompatible or unlikely with age and sex, e.g. men with cervical cancer, senile dementia in a child, testicular cancer in a woman.

This can be very time-consuming, as these searches will identify groups of patients that you will then need to review individually. However, it is quicker than reviewing all of your notes individually.

Changing information and medico-legal liability

Any of these methods may find entries that are suspected to be incorrect or incom-plete. These records would then need to be checked before the computer records are corrected or updated. Please look at your system documentation before correcting any records, as there are particular ways you should do this to lessen your medico-legal liability.

Remember that everything you do to a patient record is recorded in the audit trail. You must be able to stand up in court and explain why you changed the entry in a patient's record. If your system includes ways of changing codes that make it explicit that you are doing this to maintain accuracy you will be better off than if you have to rely on your memory.

You must remember that these checks are not infallible indicators of poor quality data. Incomplete data can simply be due to the fact that the patient has not attended the practice for their blood pressure to be recorded.

PRIMIS

By now, you are probably wondering what on earth this PRIMIS thing is. PRIMIS is a national project, funded by the NHS Information Authority. PRIMIS stands for Primary Care Information Services and the project is concerned solely with the quality of data in primary care. Generally, practices are part of a local scheme or project with their own local PRIMIS facilitator.

Contact your PCO or HA to see if there is a local scheme running. Taking part will help you sort out your data quality and in return for sending in anonymised morbidity information you will get access to extra training (usually free) and be able to compare your practice's morbidity data with all the others in the scheme, both locally and nationally.

PRIMIS uses MIQUEST to extract data from your system.[7] If you want to know more about either MIQUEST or PRIMIS have a look at the website.

WWW link   http://www.primis.nottingham.ac.uk/

 Appendix 13 is a case study about taking part in PRIMIS.

Alternatively, if there is no local PRIMIS scheme running or if you want to look just at your own data in the first instance, it is now possible, with modern reporting facilities, to do almost anything you used to have to do with MIQUEST with your own system.[20,21]

Key points

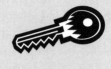

1 Quality data is complete, accurate, relevant, up to date and accessible.
2 You can find out how good you data quality is by:
   • reviewing all your notes
   • running regular reports that look at things that give you a guide to your quality
   • taking part in PRIMIS.
3 Keeping your data to a high level of quality is an ongoing commitment.

Chapter 12: Data reporting

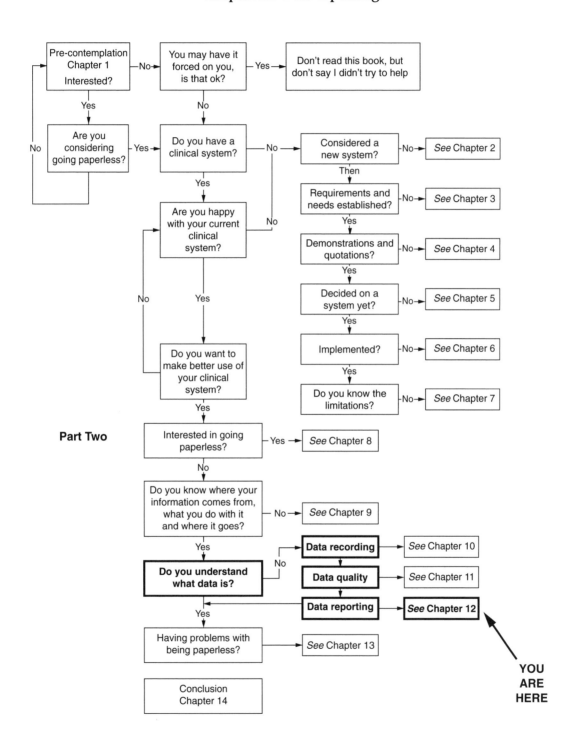

Chapter 12

Data reporting

The world is round and the place which may seem like the end may also be only the beginning.

Ivy Baker Priest 1905–75

Who should read this chapter?

You have invested a considerable amount of resources in your EPR system. You have set up data recording guidelines and are running regular reviews to check that the information being recorded is of good quality. *Finally*, you can now start to make use of your system and get some of the biggest benefits – reports!

Data reporting

As I said right at the beginning of this book, an EPR system may not help you a great deal when you have a single patient in front of you. However, where an EPR really does come into its own is reporting.

If you are consistently recording all your prescriptions, consultations and information coming in and going out of the practice you now have a wonderful source of information about your patient population that is invaluable to you.

Ad hoc requests

Just think, the next time the PCO phone you up and ask how many asthmatics you have you can answer them in seconds. All you need to do is run a report. In fact you can not only tell them how many asthmatics you have but what medication they are on and their latest PFR if the PCO really want to know!

Regular reports

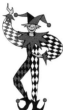All those chronic disease registers you have to keep for the NSFs are a doddle. All you need to do is set up a report that looks for the information required and run it as and when needed. There is no need for card indexes or separate databases. All the information is available from within your own EPR system. Of course, you know that the information is being recorded because as a practice you have set up templates and agreed data recording guidelines to make sure that it is.

Reports can save you time and money

So reports can save you time but what else can they do for you? They can save you money!

Savings in prescribing costs

Let's think about primary care a minute. Where do we normally try and make savings? Well, an obvious choice is prescribing. You can easily search your information to check that your patients are on the cheapest, effective medication available.

What else can you do? You can demonstrate your workload and provide evidence that you need extra staff or support. You can easily justify your need for an increase in your prescribing budgets because you can readily demonstrate that your population has a particularly high group of patients requiring expensive medications.

You can provide evidence to your local trust that you need an extra specialist in a particular area. The list is endless.

As long as you get the principles of good quality recording and consistent coding right your system will repay itself to you in kind many times over.

Key points

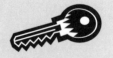

1 The biggest benefit of going paperless is everything you can achieve with searches and reports (once you have got past the initial effort of going paperless!).
2 You will save yourself time and money.

Chapter 13: Problems with being paperless

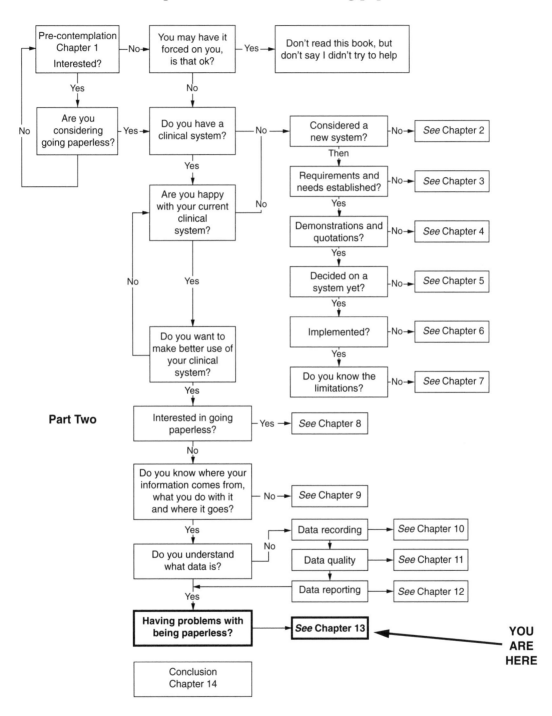

Chapter 13

Problems with being paperless

Expect trouble as an inevitable part of life and repeat to yourself the most comforting words of all: this, too, will pass.

Ann Landes 1918–

Who should read this chapter?

You have read this book and are still unsure whether or not you think that going paperless is a good idea. You have read all about the benefits of an EPR and being paperless but you want to balance the argument and think about the possible problems.

Problems

It would be wrong to suggest that there are not significant problems that you will need to deal with if you decide to go paperless. However, I will say that the known problems can be dealt with quite simply. Usually all you need is extra training and at the end of the day, do you really think that you will have a choice for much longer about using an EPR?

Coding

Until the suppliers develop systems that code for you, you will need to understand the Read codes. As I hope to have demonstrated, your information must be consistent and complete. You are actually putting your patient at risk every time you use an incorrect or illogical code. You are also increasing your medico-legal liability.

Handwriting

By using an EPR you will lose the added value that you may get from seeing your own handwriting. Many doctors agree that when they look at the last entry on the patients notes they can tell what mood they had been in at the time. If they think that they were in a bad mood that day or in a rush, they may take more time with the patient on this occasion.

Locums

Locums will need extensive training on the system and your data entry protocols. Alternatively, you will need to develop alternative ways of getting their information into your system.

Items of service (IOS)

All members of the primary care team will need to understand IOS links, as they will be generated automatically as a result of the consultation.

Power and system failures

You will experience power and system failures at some point. Your paperless world will come crashing down around your ears. Make sure that you have a contingency plan for getting information into your system.

Resource commitment

Going paperless will cost you a fortune in terms of time, money, effort, learning and cultural change. You will also need to commit a significant amount of time to keep all the IT working within you practice.

It is irreversible

The biggest problem is that once you have gone paperless, you will never want to go backwards and will wonder how you ever managed before. If you don't believe me just watch what happens when you have your first system or power failure!

Key points

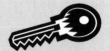

1 Going paperless will not be easy or problem-free.
2 Training will help to ease the problems considerably.
3 You will need to understand coding.
4 You will lose the value of handwritten records.
5 You will need to decide how to deal with locums and other non-primary care team data entry.
6 You will need to understand your IOS submissions.
7 Going paperless will cost you.
8 **Having said all that, once you've gone paperless you will never want to go back to a paper-based practice!**

Chapter 14: Conclusion

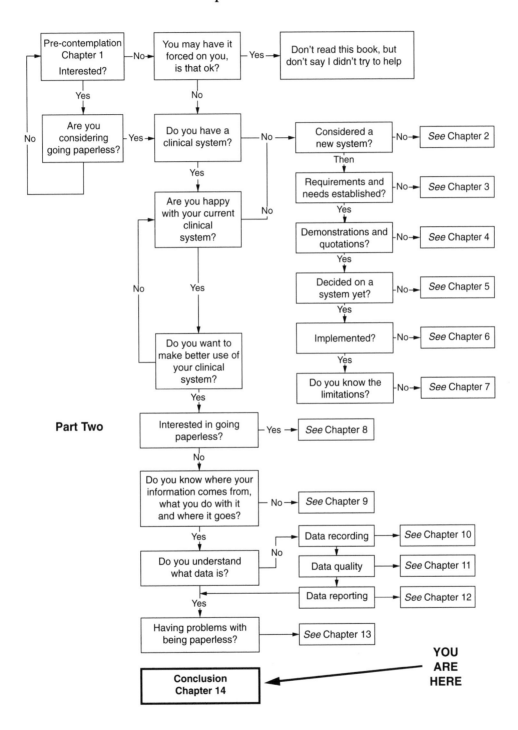

Pre-contemplation
Chapter 1
Interested?

—No→ You may have it forced on you, is that ok? —Yes→ Don't read this book, but don't say I didn't try to help

Yes

No

Are you considering going paperless? —Yes→ Do you have a clinical system? —No→ Considered a new system? —No→ *See* Chapter 2

Then

No

Requirements and needs established? —No→ *See* Chapter 3

Yes

Yes

Are you happy with your current clinical system? —No→

Demonstrations and quotations? —No→ *See* Chapter 4

Yes

No

Yes

Decided on a system yet? —No→ *See* Chapter 5

Yes

Do you want to make better use of your clinical system?

Implemented? —No→ *See* Chapter 6

Yes

Yes

Do you know the limitations? —No→ *See* Chapter 7

Part Two

Interested in going paperless? — Yes → *See* Chapter 8

No

Do you know where your information comes from, what you do with it and where it goes? — No → *See* Chapter 9

Yes

Data recording → *See* Chapter 10

Do you understand what data is? —No→ Data quality → *See* Chapter 11

Yes

Data reporting → *See* Chapter 12

Yes

Having problems with being paperless? → *See* Chapter 13

**Conclusion
Chapter 14** ← **YOU ARE HERE**

Chapter 14

Conclusion

Something which we think is impossible now is not impossible in another decade.
Constance Baker Motly 1921–

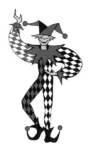

If you are still reading in an effort to cure insomnia, and the warm bath and hot milky drink didn't work, try reading all 13 appendices, glossary and index!

Seriously, if you have read and worked your way through either or both parts of this book, you will now have a primary care clinical system that does what you need it to do *and* you will be using it effectively and getting all those benefits you were promised.

Is the paperless practice a case of the Emperor's new clothes? I'll let you answer that.

Are you getting the benefits you expected of going paperless?

If the benefits of going paperless are still invisible to you, please have another look at Part Two! It will take a lot of time and effort but it is worth it. If you don't believe me, go and ask those who have tried it.

If the benefits are no longer invisible but real and helping you to do what you do best – provide good quality patient care – then please follow Pooh's advice and share your experiences with your friends and colleagues. It is only by learning from each other that we ever see real progress.

> It isn't good having anything exciting (like floods), if you can't share them with somebody.
>
> *Winnie the Pooh* AA Milne

Appendices

Appendix I
Benefits of an EPR in primary care

A number of publications state that there are many benefits of an EPR in primary care. For more information, have a look at NHS HIS Lambeth, Southwark and Lewisham's Noteless Practice Support Pack[22] or any of the papers referenced below. I am sure that this list is not comprehensive but it will give you a flavour.

Quality of care benefits

Computer-based records help clinicians by:

1   Improving the quality of and access to patient information.[23]
2   Integrating information over time and between settings of care.[23]
3   Giving decision support to practitioners.[23]
4   Helping to improve clinical practice.[24]
5   Reducing clinical errors.[25]
6   Addressing the need to record a greater quality of information.[26]
7   Encouraging a consistent approach to the management of clinical problems. [26]
8   Ensuring that essential information (chronic conditions) is highlighted through the use of automated reminders.[27]
9   Helping them to keep more complete records.[27]

Cost of care benefits

Computer-based records reduce costs by:

1 Reducing redundant tests and services due to unavailability of test results.[23]
2 Saving administration costs by generating reports automatically and electronic submission of claims.
3 Enhancing productivity by reducing:
   • the time needed to find missing records or wait for records already in use
   • redundant data entry
   • the time needed to enter or review data in seconds.[23]
4 Reducing risks to the patient (and thus unnecessary costs of care) arising out of:
   • decisions that are delayed due to inability to find/access information
   • repeating invasive tests/procedures (all procedures carry some risk of morbidity or mortality however small these risks may be)
   • minimising the probability of adverse effects or interactions arising from drugs prescribed by practitioners unaware of the full clinical situation.[23]
5 Reducing legal exposure arising out of medical records that are inadequate, incomplete or unable to be found when required.[22]
6 Reducing the likelihood of information going missing.[23]
7 Improving the security of information.[29]
8 Improving efficiency.[28,30]
9 Increasing income.[27]
10 Providing more detailed records in case of future litigation.[26]
11 Saving time producing activity information.[22]
12 Saving space by not having to store records in the reception area.[22]

Communication benefits

1 Improved access to clinical information for patients.[27]
2 Faster access to pathology and radiology results.[22]
3 Improved sharing of health information across the wide range of professionals who work in primary care.[22]
4 Improved flow of information across the interfaces with NHS trusts.[29]
5 Improved legibility of notes.[27,28]

Analysis benefits

1   Easier observation of trends and patterns in the health of a patient.[27]
2   Easier clinical audit, outcome assessment and research.[27,29]
3   Ability to analyse data to support management decision making.[26]
4   Enables the demonstration of clinical competence for revalidation purposes.[22]

Appendix 2
A buyer's checklist

Tasks

1 Establish a coordinator to oversee all aspects of computerisation.   ❑
2 Select key staff-members for participation in the planning process.   ❑
3 Engage in background reading and familiarise yourself with products available.   ❑
4 Ask your local PCO/HA if they offer assistance.   ❑
5 Review the needs of your practice.   ❑
6 Write down your major objectives for computerisation.   ❑
7 Visit colleagues' practices to review systems that have been in place for 6–12 months.   ❑
8 Establish desired time lines for each objective.   ❑
9 Regularly brief all practice staff on planning.   ❑
10 Formulate a detailed list of your requirements of a new system. The more details the better (e.g. allows the doctor to hand the script to the patient within 15 seconds of pressing the print button).   ❑
11 Investigate finance options with your financial adviser and with your PCO and HA.   ❑
12 Formulate a supplier/product shortlist.   ❑
13 Appraise the products offered by the various suppliers.   ❑
14 Formulate a 'request for proposal' or 'RFP' (based on your detailed list of requirements).   ❑
15 Circulate the RFP to your short-listed vendors.   ❑
16 Review and refine your requirements according to the responses you receive.   ❑

17 Review and refine proposals from potential suppliers. ❏
18 Document and refine a training, data transfer, implementation and support plan. ❏
19 Select computer system. ❏
20 Arrange finance. ❏
21 Formulate a payment plan that allows you to test the performance of your new system before you pay. ❏
22 Finalise a well-documented contract with your supplier that includes your requirements for the system, for training, for data transfer, for implementation and support. ❏
23 Prepare the practice and the staff for implementation. ❏
24 Arrange and plan system installation. ❏
25 Arrange for the transfer of data into the new system. ❏
26 Arrange system testing prior to final acceptance and payment. ❏
27 Finalise training for practice staff including the level of skill you expect each to attain (e.g. able to prepare script electronically without assistance). ❏
28 Document new procedures, this is often best achieved during system training. ❏
29 'D-day' – enjoy the pleasures of your new system. ❏

Source: Reproduced with permission from the GPCG Buyer's checklist. In: GPCG (1999) *Buying Computer Systems For General Practice.* Version 1.1, June.[31]
© Commonwealth of Australia, 1999

Appendix 3
GPIMM and TNAMM

Please note:
This appendix provides a brief overview of two tools that might help you identify your information and training needs. All information was correct at the time of going to press.

The information provided represents the views of the supplier, not necessarily those of the author.

Introduction

GPIMM (General Practice Information Maturity Model) and TNAMM (Training Needs Analysis Maturity Model) are tools that are designed to address the known problems with the current state of the NHS IM&T (Information Management and Technology) infrastructure, which is characterised by:

- lots of IT, little information
- incompatible systems
- little use of effective coding
- systems that sucked in data, but did not provide information.

This state of affairs has been exacerbated by a number of factors:

- lots of technology, e.g. nearly 100% of GPs are computerised, yet EHRs remain a distant dream for most in primary care

- clinicians have often been excluded from the IM&T agenda, sometimes but not always by their own choice or simply because of the pressure of other commitments
- training has been limited and piecemeal in fashion, with no links made to organisational goals
- much resource has been dedicated to expensive high tech demonstrator projects that may have a high technical content but limited clinical benefit.

In order to deliver more effective information, GPIMM and TNAMM advocate a step-by-step approach that links technology, process and training. The authors of these tools argue that there needs to be an appreciation of everyday clinical needs by IM&T staff and early delivery of clinical benefits to enthuse the sceptics.

A step-by-step approach

Information for Health defines a step-by-step approach. However, this view of the EHR is very high level and is also technology- rather than clinically-focused. From a pragmatic point of view, it's not the levels that are the problem: it's how to get from one to the next!

GPIMM (General Practice Information Maturity Model)

Background

The idea of the maturity model is based upon the capability maturity model (CMM) developed by the Software Engineering Institute (SEI) of Carnegie Mellon University. The SEI CMM was developed for the US Department of Defence to model the maturity of quality processes within their software suppliers.

The SEI maturity model is defined as a five-level framework for how an organisation matures its software processes from ad hoc, chaotic processes to mature, disciplined software processes.

SEI (1995) describes the levels as described in the table below.

The five levels of the SEI CMM

Level	Designation	Description
1	Initial	The organisation has undefined processes and controls
2	Repeatable	The organisation has standardised methods facilitating repeatable processes
3	Defined	The organisation monitors and improves its processes
4	Managed	The organisation possesses advanced controls, metrics and feedback
5	Optimising	The organisation uses metrics for optimisation purposes

Source: SEI (1995).

The SEI CMM is questionnaire-based. Questions are divided into 'essentials' and 'highly desirable'. To achieve a given level, an organisation must attain 90% 'yes' answers to essential questions and 80% 'yes' answers to highly desirable questions. The CMM has become an international standard in its field.

The CMM provides a way of telling you where you are and how to improve.

The GPIMM is derived from the CMM. The key characteristics of the SEI CMM as used in the GPIMM model are:

- recognition that change and improvement are dynamic processes
- definition of characteristics to define key stages of maturity
- definition of key actions to define how to move from each level to the next
- use of a questionnaire to facilitate analysis of current maturity.

The five levels of the GPIMM

Level	Designation	Description
0	Paper-based	The practice has no computer system
1	Computerised	The practice has a computer system. It is used only by the practice staff
2	Computerised primary healthcare team	The practice has a computer system. It is used by the practice staff and the primary healthcare team, including the doctors
3	Coded	The system makes limited use of Read codes
4	Bespoke	The system is tailored to the needs of the practice through agreed coding policies and the use of clinical protocols
5	Paperless	The practice is completely paperless, except where paper records are a legal requirement

TNAMM (Training Needs Analysis Maturity Model)

Background

A TNAMM has recently been added to the GPIMM. This is based upon the key skills and competencies that staff need to deliver the change defined by GPIMM.

The training needs tool defines need according to both organisational role and maturity. In this way, it provides a view of training need that accurately reflects the needs of the organisation at that time. Further, it may be used to predict training requirements in the light of planned organisational developments.

The result is a tool that can:

- audit practices' current information maturity
- provide practice improvement plans
- monitor actual improvements
- define competency levels for key roles
- audit staff against required competencies
- draw up training strategies tied to organisational goals
- monitor competency levels against key targets.

This is all provided within a convenient easy to use computer-based tool available in versions for Access97™ or Access2000™. For large installations, an SQL server back end is also available. However, this is rarely required.

Contact

For more information about either of these tools, please contact

Professor Alan Gillies
Professor of Information Management
Health Informatics Research Unit
University of Central Lancashire
Preston PR1 2HE

Tel: +44 1772 893870

Website: www.healthinformatics.org.uk
email: professor@alangillies.co.uk

Appendix 4
Questions to ask your staff

1   What are your main problems/complaints with our current system?
2   If we have more workstations, where should they be?
3   Do you have a computer at home? If so, do you use it yourself?
4   Would you prefer a 'Windows®'-based system to the current one?
5   Would you use the computer more if it were:
    • mouse operated?
    • voice operated?
6   If it were voice operated and easy to use, would you dictate your own letters?
7   Would it help to have a list of standard Read codes for major diseases?
8   Would you like dedicated time to learn more about your computer?
9   Do you think we need an externally taught course?
10 Do you hate your printer? Why?
11 If you could have other programmes – Office®, Publisher®, CDROM library – what would you like and would you use them?
12 What else would you like on the computer (games?)?
13 Have you used the Internet? If so, why?
    Should the practice have access to it? If so why?
14 Would you like to go 'paperless'?

Source: originally developed by and with Chelford Surgery (1999). Unpublished documentation and personal correspondence.[32]

Appendix 5
An overview of EMIS, In Practice Systems and Torex Health

Please note:
This appendix provides a brief overview of some of the information you will need to know about each of the suppliers when you are considering buying one of their systems. All information was correct at the time of going to press.

The suppliers are dealt with in alphabetical order and the information provided represents the views of the suppliers, not necessarily those of the author.

EMIS

> *EMIS takes care of its practices.*
> Dr David Stables, Interview 10 May 2001

Company history

Egton Medical Information Systems Ltd was founded by Dr Peter Sowerby (Chairman), Mr Tony Jones (Managing Director) and Dr David Stables (Medical Director) in 1987. The original system was based on a system developed within a dispensing practice in Egton near Whitby in the 1980s. The company is privately owned and Sean Riddell (Deputy MD) has recently joined the board of directors.

Over 4700 general practices within the UK use EMIS. EMIS is also used by homeless health projects in London, drug dependency units, hospices and community health professionals.

Company policy

EMIS have remained independent and have grown organically without acquisition of other primary care companies. They focus almost entirely on primary care with some overlap with community care. They collaborate extensively with secondary care to ensure system integration and connectivity as required. Their system is used in a small number of secondary care settings including a long-term stay and community hospital.

Purchasing an EMIS system

Timing

At the moment it will take about 8–10 weeks from your decision to purchase an EMIS system to having it installed in your premises. This time varies according to demand. It will be about 18 months before your relationship with EMIS will be simply one of ongoing maintenance and support. This is because they provide a lot of extra support and assistance over the first year after implementation.

Costs

Like most clinical systems EMIS does not have a price list that you can just pick and choose from. Costs will be determined by your individual requirements. As a rough guide, costs are generally calculated pro rata to the number of GPs in you practice.

Hardware

EMIS will not force you to buy your hardware from them though they are often quite competitive with high street prices. There is an exception to this. You *must* buy your server from EMIS, which will be provided with smart UPS as standard.

Data conversion

All data conversions are undertaken in-house by a department of about 16 people. EMIS are very confident of converting data successfully from the majority of suppliers. However, if you have a home grown system, or one where the user base is fewer than 50, do allow extra time as this will prove more difficult.

Codes

The majority of EMIS sites are using version 2 (5-byte) of the Read codes with about 60 practices still on version 1 (4-byte). Having had a hiatus for a while, EMIS are now happily converting practices from version 1 to version 2 if they choose to do so.

If you purchase an EMIS system today it will use version 2 of the Read codes (5 byte).

EMIS use their own drug database, which is RFA99 compliant and incorporates the BNF drug data on licence. In addition to the Read codes, you will find there are a number of EMIS codes used within the system. Do watch out for these.

Free text
If you have free text *associated with a code* in your current system, EMIS will be able to import this into their system.

Installation
Installation is usually completed in one day, though it has been known to take two for very complex situations.

Training
EMIS provides different types of training. They can provide a lot on site for you. Additionally, they have a training suite that is also used. When you buy an EMIS system you will receive validated training in all the modules you buy as well as general Windows® training, if required.

Post installation

System maintenance
EMIS is designed so that it automatically validates and re-indexes on a weekly basis. Additionally, EMIS provides a dial-in service known as the 'Patch' system to their users. This service is used to provide all upgrades and support. About two-thirds of EMIS users use this Patch system on NHSnet with the remainder using it via direct asynchronous dial-up via the practice modem.

Upgrades
It is EMIS policy that all new software developments, enhancements and upgrades are provided *free of charge* to all users.

Support
EMIS engineers are based in the field so can be with you fairly quickly if you do have a problem. However, the vast majority of software problems can be dealt with over the Patch system.

EMIS

EMIS has two systems:

1 **EMIS LV**, which is a text-based system running on a combination platform of M and Delphi with the ability to run in a Windows NT® and Windows 2000®, environment.

2 **EMIS GV** running in Windows 2000® using a Microsoft SQL® Server as the back end database.

Both systems include integrated appointment systems. There is also a portable version of EMIS that allows you to download copies of a small selection of your patient records for use on home visits.

EMIS clinical system components

1 Patient management.
2 Intelligent prescribing.
3 Consultation mode.
4 Dispensing.
5 Communications.
6 Appointments.
7 MENTOR (EMIS' clinical information and knowledge support system for GPs).
8 Patient information leaflets (PILs).
9 Classification (Read codes and EMIS' own drug database).
10 Word processor.
11 Formulary management.
12 Electronic *BNF*.
13 PRODIGY.
14 Electronic health record communicator.

Data recording

EMIS comes with standard templates and protocols. These can be edited or new ones created by users. EMIS also has a facility called quick key, which lets you automate data entry tasks by assigning a set of actions to a 'quick key'. This is often used to speed up prescribing.

Data reporting

EMIS has a search and statistics module that allows users to run both very simple searches and complex audits. System audits are included for a variety of subjects including health promotion, cytology and immunisation.

EDI

Registration and IOS are available for all practices. Over 1800 practices are also using GP/laboratory links.

Why you should buy EMIS

The breadth of EMIS' system functionality is greater than most. The majority of people find it is much easier to use and we are more consistent than most. Our five-year ownership costs are significantly less than others. The system design is very strongly influenced by the National User Group.

Dr David Stables, Interview 10 May 2001

Contact details

Administration, sales and marketing, software support and development personnel are based in Leeds, as are the communications and hardware engineering divisions.

Training is regionalised and headed by regional operations directors and their deputies. The regional managers manage teams of operations managers who provide high levels of local area support and contact. The total compliment of staff employed by EMIS is around 560.

EMIS Head Office
Park House Mews
77 Back Lane
Horsforth
Leeds
LS18 4RF

EMIS Town Street Office
57/59 Town Street
Horsforth
Leeds LS18 5BP

Administration
  Tel: 0113 259 1122
  email: emis@e-mis.com

Training helpline
  Tel: 08701 221133
  email: support@e-mis.com

Sales and Marketing
  Tel: 0113 297 4470
  email: sales@e-mis.com

Support
  email: support@e-mis.com

Central operations
  Tel: 0113 297 4490
  email: centraloperations@e-mis.com

WWW link   http://www.emis-online.com/

In Practice Systems

Vision is <u>the</u> premiere Windows GP system
Dr Mike Robinson, Interview 1 May 2001

Company history

In Practice Systems Ltd can be traced back to the early 1980s when Value Added Medical Products (VAMP) was formed. In the early 1990s VAMP became part of Reuters until 1998, when the European health businesses of Reuters were acquired by the Cegedim group. At this time the company was re-launched as In Practice Systems (IPS). The Cegedim group is the leading supplier of clinical management systems throughout Europe.

Vision is currently the most widely used Windows® clinical management system with over 1500 sites in UK primary care.

Company policy

IPS is committed to industry open platforms; they are a Microsoft Certified Partner. They are primarily focused on providing an integrated system for primary and community care providers; they collaborate extensively with secondary care to ensure system integration and connectivity as required.

Purchasing Vision

Timing
At the moment it will take about 8–10 weeks from your decision to purchase a VISION system to having it installed in your premises. It will be about 12 months before your relationship with IPS will be simply one of ongoing maintenance and support. This is because they provide a lot of extra support and assistance over the first year after implementation.

Costs
The costs of a Vision implementation will be determined by your individual requirements. As a rough guide, costs are generally calculated pro rata to the number of workstations you will need in your practice.

Hardware
IPS will not force you to buy your hardware from them though they are often quite competitive with high street prices. There is an exception to this. They will *strongly* encourage you to buy your server from IPS, which will be provided with UPS as standard.

Data conversion

Data conversions are undertaken by a combination of in-house staff and third party companies. Data extraction from other systems is primarily undertaken by third party companies with IPS undertaking the importation of this data into Vision themselves. They are very confident of converting data successfully from the majority of suppliers. Occasionally, if you only have a home-grown system or very little data to convert, you may prefer to start with a clean system, just importing your patient details from a health authority download.

Codes

Vision primarily uses version 2 (5 byte) of the Read codes. Additionally, as Vision offer a lot of support for community care staff you will find that there are a large number of Read Version 3 terms included, as user-defined codes to support community working.

Vision uses Multilex as its drug dictionary.

Free text

If you have free text *associated with a code* in your current system, IPS will be able to import this into Vision.

Installation

Installation is managed by an in-house engineering team who will install and configure the system and verify that your converted data has been correctly loaded.

Training

IPS provides different types of training. They can provide a lot on site for you. When you buy a Vision system you will receive a minimum of five days training. However, they do recommend that at least ten days training is required to really make sure that you have covered all the modules, as well as general Windows® training.

Post installation

System maintenance

IPS provides dial-in support over NHSnet for system maintenance.

Upgrades

Currently IPS sends out all upgrades on CDROM, but from late 2001, IPS will introduce an upgrade distribution service utilising practice NHSnet connections as they are activated. It is IPS policy that all new software enhancement and upgrades are provided *free of charge* to all users.

Support

IPS engineers are based in the field so can be with you fairly quickly if you do have a problem.

In Practice Systems

IPS has a single full Windows®-based system.

Vision (running in Windows NT®). This includes an integrated appointment system.

Vision clinical system components
1 Clinical records.
2 EDI messaging.
3 Appointments.
4 Searches and reports.
5 Prescribing decision support and PRODIGY.
6 Clinical audit and data extraction.
7 User definable clinical guidelines.

Data recording
Vision comes with standard templates and protocols. These can be edited or new ones created by users. Vision also has a facility called Snapcards, which provides you with current and historical information in a clear grid format, which assists with clinical management.

Data reporting
Vision has extensive in-built searching and reporting capabilities. The clinical audit module allows users to run both very simple searches and complex audits easily.

EDI
Registration, IOS and GP provider links are available for all practices.

Why you should buy VISION

Vision is the premiere Windows GP system that supports the whole of primary care. It is a mature product, well established in the market and is continually evolving and being updated. Its foremost position in the Windows arena means it is the most complete solution, without question.

Dr Mike Robinson, Interview 1 May 2001

Contact details

IPS Head Office
The Bread Factory
1a Broughton Street
London SW8 3QJ

IPS Training Office
Shillingwood House
Westwood Way
Westwood Business Park
Coventry CV4 8JZ

Tel: 0207 501 7000
Fax: 0207 501 7100
General sales enquires:
   sales@inps.co.uk

Tel: 024 7642 2334
Fax: 024 7647 1662

WWW link   http://www.inps.co.uk/

Torex Health

Designed by clinicians, for clinicians.
Dr Mike Bainbridge, Interview 17 May 2001

Company history

Torex Health Ltd was formed in January 2000 following a merger between Torex Medical and Torex Meditel, creating the fastest growing company in the UK clinical systems market. Torex Health has brought together many systems and users with a wealth of diverse experience over more than 20 years.

Torex Health is a wholly owned subsidiary of Torex PLC. Torex Health provides integrated solutions and supporting services across the acute, community and primary care sectors. They aim to meet all the clinical and administrative needs across the continuum of care, including the implementation of an Electronic Health Record (EHR).

Company policy

Unlike EMIS and IPS, Torex Health does not focus only on primary and community care systems. Torex Health has the largest hospital information system client base in the UK, supplies pathology and radiology solutions and can provide fully outsourced solutions.

Torex Health are positioning themselves to provide integrated clinical solutions across the continuum of care including PCTs.

Purchasing Torex Health

Timing

At the moment it will be about 8–10 weeks from your decision to purchase a Torex Health system to having it installed in your premises.

It will be about 12 months before your relationship with Torex Health will be simply one of ongoing maintenance and support. This is because they provide a lot of extra support and assistance over the first year after implementation.

Costs

Like most clinical systems Torex Health does not have a price list that you can just pick and choose from. Costs will be determined by your individual requirements. As a rough guide, costs are generally calculated pro rata to the number of GPs in your practice and the number of workstations.

Hardware

Torex Health will not force you to buy your hardware from them though they are often quite competitive with high street prices. There is an exception to this. They will insist on you buying your server from Torex Health, which will be provided with UPS as standard.

Data conversion

Data conversion is undertaken in-house. They are very confident of converting data successfully from the majority of suppliers. However, if you have a home-grown system, or one where the user base is fewer than 50, do allow extra time as this will prove more difficult.

Codes

New Torex Health systems use version 2 (5 byte) of the Read codes. A significant minority of existing users are still using version 1 (4 byte) Read codes.

Torex Health System 6000 and Premiere both use the Multilex drug dictionary. This is updated monthly, and provides interaction, sensitivity and allergy checking.

Free text

If you have free text associated with a code in your current system Torex Health will be able to import this into System 6000 and Premiere.

Installation

Installation is usually completed in one day, although it has been known to take two for very complex situations.

Training

Torex Health provides different types of training. They can provide a lot on site for you. When you buy a Torex Health system you will receive validated training in all the modules you buy.

Additionally, there is extensive online help and even some computer-based training for some of the applications.

Advanced training on reports and SOPHIE template writing is also available

Post installation

System maintenance

Currently, practice staff must undertake system maintenance and upgrades manually. Torex Health sends out all upgrades on CDROM. However, increasing use is made of the practices' NHSnet connection to supply patches and provide technical support.

Upgrades

It is Torex Health policy to supply standard software enhancements and upgrades *free of charge* to all users.

Support

Torex Health provides a field staff of specially trained engineers, covering all areas of the UK. The vast majority of software problems can be resolved remotely over BT line or NHSnet by the support desk without recourse to engineers.

Torex Health

Torex has three RFA99 accredited systems and one in the accreditation process.

1 **Torex Premiere** is an easy to use Windows NT®- or UNIX®-based solution developed for clinicians by clinicians.
2 **Torex System 6000** was the first system in the UK to meet the RFA 99 accreditation and provides a comprehensive problem-orientated solution, using Windows® on NT® and UNIX®.
3 **Visual Phenix** is a fully functional Windows®-based solution used predominantly in the Pennines.
4 **System 5** is a text-based system utilised comprehensively across its large installed base.

All systems include integrated appointment systems. There is also a portable version (using palmtops) for Torex Health systems that allow you to download parts of a selection of your patient records for use on home visits. Torex's strategy is to bring these solutions together to provide a single scalable solution for GPs and PCTs alike.

Torex Health clinical system components
1 Clinical records.
2 Prescription records.
3 Integrated appointments.
4 Clinical governance and data extraction, using MIQUEST (for anonymised patient data extraction) and PRODIGY (for prescribing decision support).
5 NHSnet desktop connectivity, including EDI messaging and pathology links.
6 Palmtop (portable patient care for home visits).
7 SOPHIE (electronic clinical guidelines).
8 Anatomical drawings.
9 Reports.
10 Practice agreed formularies.
11 Automated referral letters.
12 Links to Microsoft Office suite if required.
13 Support for NSFs.

Data recording
All Torex Health Windows systems come with standard templates and protocols, which are designed for rapid data entry. These can be edited or new ones created by users and they allow users to add their own macros and shortcut keys to speed data entry.

Data reporting
Torex Health has extensive in-built searching and reporting capabilities allowing users to run both very simple searches and complex audits easily.
Standard reports are available to generate target claim information, and assist with call and recall of at-risk patients.

EDI
Registration, items of service and GP/Laboratory links are available for all practices.

Why you should buy Torex Health

All Torex systems are well established products that fully support the administration and clinical aspects of the practice. They are feature rich, support problem orientation, are very easy to use with extensive powerful reporting facilities and will continue to meet your practice IT needs in the future.

Dr Mike Bainbridge, Interview 17 May 2001

Contact details

Torex Health Ltd
Orchard House
Newton Road
Bromsgrove B60 3EA

Main switchboard: 01527 579414
Support centre: 01527 574888
Fax (general):   01527 574061
Sales office: 0114 2092661
Sales fax: 0114 2092634

General sales enquires: sales.health@torex.com
Non-urgent support enquiries: support@torexhealth.co.uk
Issues relating to the website: webmaster@torexhealth.co.uk

WWW link   http://www.torexhealth.co.uk/

Appendix 6
Request for a proposal

A request for a proposal (RFP) should contain the following sections. Be as detailed as you possibly can.

Covering statement
This first section should give the supplier details of who they should contact at the practice and any deadline you have chosen for the proposal to be sent to you.

Description of the practice
You need to provide a broad overview of your practice. You must include the number of staff and GPs, if you have a branch surgery, a description of the buildings and any existing systems.

Requirements specification
This is when you give the supplier that long detailed list of needs you agreed. Remember to give them the prioritised and latest version.

Method of evaluation
You may choose to tell the suppliers what you will be assessing them on. It may well be that particular functions, ease of use, adequate training or price are far more important to you than anything else.

Details required
Don't forget to include a list of any specific questions you want the supplier to answer. For example, you may like to ask about:

- software required (number of licences)
- hardware required (computers, wiring, furniture)
- system documentation (manuals for system use and maintenance)
- maintenance and ongoing costs (specifics of what is covered and what isn't – including response times – and what may have to be purchased later)
- training (how much, how long will it take? On the job or off-site, classroom or demonstrations)
- implementation (timetable of implementation process)
- ongoing support (arrangements for troubleshooting and advanced training).

Cost

Be very specific about how you want the costs to be detailed. If you insist that the suppliers list each purchase component separately it will make it easier for you to compare proposals from different suppliers. Do ask for as much detail as possible.

Required conditions of purchase

Don't forget that you are potentially spending a lot of money with these suppliers. Give them details of any requirements you have for the system to be fully functional and working before you will agree final payments.

Suggested configuration

Give the supplier a description of what you think are the most likely requirements. Include the number of users and the main tasks they will do. This should allow suppliers to propose alternative configurations or amendments if necessary.

Source: Reproduced with permission from GPCG (1999) *Buying Computer Systems For General Practice*. Version 1.1, June.[10]
© Commonwealth of Australia, 1999

Appendix 7
Questions to ask the suppliers

Clinical system

1 Do you include an integrated clinic appointments system (not just a diary)?
2 Does your system allow multi-user access to one record at the same time?
3 Can the user choose not to use the mouse but to use hot or quick keys instead?
4 Does the system allow easy integration with standard software such as Word and Excel?
5 Is the software intuitive to use?
6 Is the system supported by on screen context sensitive help?
7 Does the system have an online manual?

Prescribing

1 Is prescribing supported by a practice formulary?
2 Can GPs use their own drug formulary, which forms part of a practice formulary?
3 Is the system supplied with an independent online drug dictionary?
4 Is the dictionary updated monthly, without fail?
5 Does the system support dispensing practices? If so, does the system include stock control systems and/or electronic stock ordering from a variety of suppliers?

Telemedicine

Is the system capable of storing digital images in the patient record?

Upgrades

1   How often do you provide upgrades for your system?
2   Do you provide major upgrades to your system free of charge?

PRODIGY and MIQUEST

1   How compatible is PRODIGY within your system?
2   How compatible is MIQUEST within your system?

Branch surgeries

Does the system support branch surgeries? If so, how?

Links

1   Does your system support the EDI GP Links Registration service?
2   Does your system support the EDI IOS service?
3   Does your system support the EDI pathology service?
    Are EDI pathology results stored in the patient record? If so, does this require doctor authorisation or does it happen automatically?
4   Does your system support the EDI radiology service?
    Are EDI radiology results stored in the patient record? If so, does this require doctor authorisation or does it happen automatically?

Email and Internet

1   Does your system have a fully integrated X400 connection?
2   Does it provide secure X400 email to all desktops?
3   Does it provide SMTP email to all desktops?

4   Does it provide Web browsing to all desktops?
5   Does your system provide a practice intranet?

NHSnet

1   How many practices do you have linked to NHSnet? What problems have you encountered?
2   Do you provide secure support for your system through NHSnet?
3   Do you, as a company, have your own NHSnet connection?
4   Do you provide virus protection as part of your system?

Security

1   Do you invoke maximum-security options for your practice systems connected to NHSnet?
2   Do you have a practice security policy?

Hardware

1   Do you provide hardware at high street prices?
2   Can I choose to get my hardware from an alternative supplier (including or excluding the server)?

Maintenance and support

1   Do you insist that you provide hardware maintenance for all hardware?
2   Do you provide onsite hardware support within eight hours?
3   Have you ever had to refund due to failure to perform to contract?
4   Can you provide on-site hardware support within four hours if required?
5   Does the initial hardware maintenance quoted run for the full 12 months? What is the likely increase for year two and beyond?
6   Do you provide 365-/6-day, 24-hour manned cover on your support lines? If not, what do you provide?

What are your annual support charges for:

- clinical system
- appointments system
- Read codes
- drug dictionary
- registration links
- IOS links
- pathology links
- radiology links
- operating system
- server
- workstations/terminals?

Data conversion

What happens to my free text when you convert my data?

Searching and reporting

1 Can I search on anything?
2 Can I combine searches?
3 Is there anything that I can enter in the system that I can not then get back out again?

Source: These questions were originally developed by and with Chelford Surgery (1999). Unpublished documentation and personal correspondence.[32]

Appendix 8
A hardware comparison worksheet

Complete one worksheet for each supplier

Supplier:
Contact details:
Date:
Price:

CPU
Central Processing Unit – the 'brain' of the computer. Measuring speed – calculations per second:

Pentium ❑
MMX ❑ speed .... mHz
Celeron ❑
Pentium II ❑
Pentium III ❑
Xeon ❑
Atheron ❑
Other (specify) ❑

Cache
Memory used by the CPU to hold data before processing:

None ❑
128k ❑
256k ❑
512k ❑

Motherboard   *This is the 'foundation' into which drives, cards, CPU, RAM and*
               other components are added:
               Intel bx   ❏   other   ....
               Intel lx   ❏

RAM   *Fast access memory used like a 'desktop' - the more you have the*
               more files you can open at once:
               32 mb   ❏   RAM speed
               64 mb   ❏   66 mHz   ❏
               128 mb   ❏   100 mHz   ❏

Hard drive   *Your computer's 'filing cabinet'. Files are stored here when not in use*
               and when the computer is off. Files are moved from here into RAM
               when in use:
               Type
               EIDE   ❏
               SCSI   ❏   Size   .... gb

Monitor   *The screen that is used to display information:*
               Screen size   ....   Screen definition   .... dpi

Graphics adaptor *A special purpose component in the computer that is used to do all the*
               'computing' required to put pictures on the monitor screen, leaving
               your CPU to do other things:
               Type
               PCI   ❏   Graphics memory   .... mb
               AGP   ❏

CD ROM   IDE   ❏   speed   .... spin
               SCSI   ❏

Case type   *The 'box' the computer is made in. Think about where the computer*
               will sit, e.g. floor or desktop. Also contains the power supply:
               Desktop   ❏   Power supply .... watts
               Mini tower   ❏
               Full tower   ❏

Expansion slots *Various cards, or components, require 'slots' inside the computer.*
               Spare slots means the capacity to add cards (e.g. sound, graphics,
               network) at some time in the future:
               ISA free   ❏
               ISA used   ❏
               PCI free   ❏
               PCI used   ❏

Removable storage	*Large capacity drives or tapes that can be removed and stored separately to preserve data:* Tape ❑ Capacity .... mb Zip ❑ Jazz ❑ Other ❑
Modem	*Allowing your computer to 'talk' to other computers across telephone lines. Required for email and* www: Internal ❑ Speed External ❑ 28.8 kb/s ❑ 33.6 kb/s ❑ 56 k ❑

Other parts

Sound card	❑	Type	....
Floppy drive	❑	Cables	❑
Mouse	❑	Disks	❑
Mouse pad	❑	Tapes	❑
Keyboard	❑	Power filter/UPS	❑
Other		....	

Warranty *This is perhaps the most important part of your purchase. Ask questions: Where will the computer be fixed? How quickly will parts be supplied?*

Parts .... yrs
Labour .... yrs
On site ❑
Insured ❑ (Will the warranty stand if this supplier goes broke?)

Bundled software *Software that is included in the purchase price of the computer. This will include the operating system but may also include other software:*

Windows 95	❑	Microsoft Office	❑
Windows 98	❑	Anti-virus	❑
Windows NT	❑		
		Other (specify)	

Source: Reproduced with permission from GPCG (1999) *Buying Computer Systems For General Practice.* Version 1.1, June.[33]
© Commonwealth of Australia, 1999

Appendix 9
A contract checklist

Regardless of whether or not the PCO or HA take the lead on the contractual and legal parts of purchasing a system you must check that you are happy with the contract before it is signed and finally agreed. There are a number of things you should look for specifically.

Questions

1. Does the contract include a clear, fixed price for the completed work? ❏
2. Does the contract include detailed specifications of the work that is to be completed? ❏
3. Does the contract include a detailed timetable for the completion of all work, including both installation and training? ❏
4. Does the contract include a detailed schedule of payments based on the timetable for completed work? Will you have adequate opportunity to check the completed work? ❏
5. Does the contract include the provision of adequate documentation for the new system? ❏
6. Does your ongoing service agreement include arrangements for disaster recovery? Does this include a guaranteed response time when you have problems? ❏
7. Does the contract include provision for you to access software source code if your software vendor ceases operation? ❏

8   Does your contract guarantee upgrades for a specified period?   ❑

9   Are any special arrangements or verbal agreements made between
    you and the supplier included in the written contract?   ❑

Source: These questions are reproduced with permission from GPCG (1999) *Buying Computer Systems For General Practice*. Version 1.1, June.[11]
© Commonwealth of Australia, 1999

Appendix 10
Security policy

This security policy is based on a number on documents including Rhyddings Surgery and Shadsworth Surgery (2000/2001) *Beacon Information: why go paperless?*[34]

Protecting information

1   You have a duty to keep patient information confidential at all times. Be discreet.
2   Keep passwords to yourself and change them when the computer asks you to do so. Do not write them down on a Post-it note and stick to the monitor!
3   Anybody using a screen in reception must log out before leaving the screen.
4   Blank the screen between patients. It is a breach of confidentiality for the previous patient's notes to be on the screen when the next patient comes in.
5   Shred confidential printouts.
6   Insist on authorisation and identification before giving out any patient information.
7   Don't leave discs, faxes, tapes or printouts lying around.
8   Don't assume that because it is on the computer it is correct.
9   Do not leave your computer logged on when you have finished with it.

Protecting your network

1 Only your network administrator should be able to alter network connections, printers or network access.
2 The Clinical Server must be protected by password access at minimum.
3 You must use your own password. NEVER use somebody else's.
4 There must be a firewall between the clinical data and NHSnet.
5 Patient identifiable data should NOT be sent unless encrypted as agreed between the professionals and the NHS Executive.
6 All data/files that are sent or received MUST be scanned by up-to-date virus scanners.
7 Do not assume that anybody who rings up and asks for information over a network has any right or need to see it. If in doubt, just say NO.

Backup

1 Backup tapes/CD ROMS must be used in rotation, as agreed. They must be stored securely (off site) away from heat, water, cables, TVs or any other electronic or magnetic equipment.
2 Validate your backups.
3 Do not forget to backup other equipment if necessary (e.g. ECG or spirometry).
4 Don't misuse floppy discs, CD ROMS and tapes. They do not like heat or magnets.

Viruses

Viruses are small pieces of software (programmes) usually hidden within what appears to be a normal piece of software (such as email). They can damage your systems and data. They are like biological viruses in that:

- they are infectious, spreading from one machine to another on networks
- they can remain hidden for ages before becoming active
- they can kill your system – by deleting all your data, or simply changing it.

1 Keep your virus software up to date.
2 Check every disc or CD ROM that comes into the practice, no matter where it has come from (including yourself if you have used a disc at home).
3 Make sure that a virus guard programme is running on any machine that is used for email or accessing the internet/NHSnet.

4 Do not use any non-standard software (from friends, universities, etc.).
5 Do not panic if you think you have a virus:
   • STOP
   • do not let anybody use your computer
   • call for help NOW
   • follow the instructions you are given
   • do NOT switch the computer off and reboot it unless you are specifically told to do so.

Legal requirements

1 Check that your practice is registered under the Data Protection Act 1998 and that the registration details are kept up to date.
2 Data must only be disclosed to the right people.
3 Every attempt must be made to ensure that data is accurate and up to date.
4 Requests for personal data must be dealt with promptly.
5 Don't use any software unless you have a valid licence for it.
6 Make sure your computers are positioned so that the information displayed is not on public display.

Appendix 11
26 weeks to using computers in GP and practice nurse consultations

This programme was designed to help GPs and nurses who do not yet use their practice computer during consultations. It is based on research (for a Psychology Masters degree) and has been replicated from the Noteless Practice Support Pack developed by the NHS Health Informatics Service; Lambeth, Southwark and Lewisham.[16]

Week	Training needs and activities
1	**Training need: selecting patients and accessing a consultation screen** Call up and check the existing computer records of each patient prior to/during the consultation. Begin with one or two patients, and add more during each session. Do not attempt to make any entries.
2–3	**Training need: adding acute prescriptions and printing prescriptions/ adding nursing procedures** Enter acute prescriptions (doctors and prescribing nurses) or procedures (non-prescribing nurses) for the last patient in each session. If the last patient does not need medication/treatment, enter the details of an earlier patient after the last patient has left the room. In week 3, begin printing the prescriptions.

Week	Training needs and activities

4–12 Training need: using formularies, changing to and from generics
Enter prescription/procedure for second last and last patient, then third to last to last patients, etc., initially at a rate of one extra patient every week. Gradually increase the number of extra patients each week, until the above information is being entered for all patients. Working 'backwards' prevents knock-on delays occurring early in consultation sessions. The time spent during this period will improve speed and confidence so do not cut this short unless you are impatient to proceed.

13–14 Training need: repeat prescribing
Update repeat prescribing when these are changed (week 13) and begin printing them (week 14). Combine these two steps when you understand how to print selected items only, and how to cancel items selected in error.

15–16 Training need: recording non-Read code entries (e.g. blood pressure readings, weights and heights)
Add any examination findings, ensuring that all blood pressures are added for the first two days, then add additional findings in stages.

17–19 Training need: diagnoses/symptoms and where to use Read codes
In addition to the above, begin entering the reason for the consultation. You need to understand Read codes and their hierarchies. In week 19, begin entering missing historical records of major significance as you encounter them.

20–22 Training need: using disease-specific screens (e.g. diabetes)
Once the above standard has been achieved, begin using additional consultation screens. Familiarise yourself with one thoroughly. And find out whether records entered here appear on different screens or whether they will subsequently only be accessed through this one. Then progress to using other screens, but not until you are confident with using the first one.

23–25 Training need: searches and recalls
Start adding one additional screening item per week for appropriate consultations (e.g. blood pressure in week 22, blood pressure plus smoking in week 23, etc.).

Week	Training needs and activities
26	**Training need: routine troubleshooting (e.g. dealing with frozen screens)** After six months, each of the doctors and nurses should be capable of updating consultation details efficiently and managing their own systems to a reasonable level. On going training in advanced features and shortcuts will be required, as will upgrade training when new software or hardware is installed. Once all consultation details are being entered, as well as tests and investigations and correspondence from external sources, reliance on manual records will diminish and these can stop being used. Records will occasionally be needed to refer to historical items of correspondence, but will not be needed to be pulled routinely for all consultations.

Source: Applebee K (2001) 26 weeks to using computers in GP and practice nurse consultations. In: NHS HIS Lambeth, Southwark and Lewisham (2001) Noteless Practice Support Pack: a resource for GP practices.

Appendix 12
Read codes

Introduction

Read codes are a coded thesaurus of clinical terms, which enable you to make effective use of your computer systems. The codes make it easier to access information within patient records. This makes reporting, auditing, research, automating repetitive tasks, electronic communication and decision support much easier.

Whether we like them or not, codes are here to stay.

Background

Read codes are named after Dr James Read who used to be a GP. The Read clinical codes were sold to the Crown for £1.25 million and made the de facto standard for primary care computerisation in the late 1980s (now a formalised standard through RFA).

Why do we need a thesaurus of codes?

Competent computer programs can search for anything that has been typed into it. However, typing mistakes, different words for the same thing and other human foibles mean that it can be very difficult to be sure that what you find is what you meant.

So something is needed that will reduce these errors. That 'something' is clinical coding. Searching a database (of patients' illnesses or medication) for a particular code is much quicker than looking in the written notes.

Ideally, codes should be automatically and invisibly added to freely typed (free text) entries but there are a lot of technical difficulties associated with this. As a result, most clinical computer systems will expect you to select a code yourself. However all Read codes have terms associated with them. This term (an accompanying string of text known as the 'rubric') is often the phrase you would use yourself.

It is important to try to conform to any coding practices in your practice. You should at least try to code any new significant diagnoses. For instance, diabetes and asthma codes are important because they are used to recruit for relevant clinics, and to collect figures for your practice report. Contraception codes might be used for IOS claims. Anything, which would be written on the summary card in the paper record, should be recorded in the computerised medical record as a Read code. Some systems have the ability to create new 'practice' codes for use when you can't find a suitable one within Read. These codes cannot be communicated outside the practice (if you ever wanted to) because they are unique to that site.

Confused? You soon will be!

The idea is relatively simple but the reality is not. There are several versions of Read codes out there in general practice. Read version 3 is the successor to Read version 2, which comes in two versions, either 4-byte Read 4, or its successor 5-byte Read 5. **Pay attention!** Read version 3.0 has been abandoned and the version released is 3.1.

Read version 1? Don't ask!

Read 3.1 has not been taken up by any GP suppliers to date, only hospitals. So the idea of anyone being able to talk to anyone else is still a pipe dream!

Version 2 of the Read codes is complex in itself. It is based on a hierarchy of codes, which in itself causes problems – for example there are different codes for pneumoccal meningitis depending on whether it is considered an infectious or neurological condition.

Read 3 gets round this problem by losing the hierarchical coding structure. Take it from professional coders that this a good move.

There are other inconsistencies: the absence of, for instance, a code for 'unemployed' in Chapter 0 'occupations', perhaps reflecting political influence on the NHS-funded institution. 'Unemployed' is found in Chapter 1 'History/symptoms' as is 'university student'. 'University teacher' being an occupation is in Chapter 0.

Of course, these idiosyncrasies are not too apparent during consultations but difficulties with coding sometimes are. In version 2 (Read 4 and 5) there are too many codes for depression, none of which appropriately code mild depression but Read version 3.1 does deal with this.

When you have time to do so and a system that allows it, it's worth exploring the Read codes. Do this by selecting a dummy patient;[†] most systems have one and going up to the top level or chapter headings of the code (*see* chapter headings list below). From here, you can choose a branch and follow it down. Like browsing through a textbook or the yellow pages of the telephone directory, you may find something of interest. Even if you do not, it will demonstrate to you the structure of the system. Don't worry that Read 3 doesn't use the hierarchical system – just understand the idea.

The chapter headings in version 2 are shown below.

Numeric = processes of care

(Encompasses: symptoms, signs, investigations, procedures and administration)

Chapter name	Chapter number
Occupations	0
History/symptoms	1
Examination/signs	2
Diagnostic procedures	3
Laboratory procedures	4
Radiology/physics in medicine	5
Preventive procedures	6
Operations and procedures	7
Other therapeutic procedures	8
Administration	9

Capital letter = diagnoses, Lower case letter = drugs

Chapter name	Chapter letter	Chapter name	Chapter letter
Infectious/parasitic diseases	A	Gastro/intestinal system	a
Neoplasms	B	Cardiovascular system	b
Endocrine/metabolic diseases	C	Respiratory system	c
Blood disease	D	Central nervous system	d
Mental disorders	E	Infections	e

cont.

[†]**'Which of your patients is a dummy?'** Try Mr M Mouse, J Bloggs, Mr Test and Mr Dummy ...

Chapter name	Chapter letter	Chapter name	Chapter letter
Nervous system/sense diseases	F	Endocrine system	f
Circulatory system diseases	G	Obst/gynae/urinary tract	g
Respiratory system disease	H	Malignant disease and immunosuppressant	h
Digestive system diseases	I	Nutrition and blood	i
Genito-urinary diseases	J	Musculoskeletal/Joint	j
Preg/childbirth/puerperium	K	Eye drugs	k
Skin/subcutaneous tissue diseases	L	Ear, nose and oropharnyx	l
Musculoskeletal diseases	M	Skin	m
Congenital anomalies	N	Immunology	n
Perinatal anomalies	O	Anaesthesia	o
Injury and poisoning	P	Appliances and reagents	p
Causes of injury and poisoning	Q	Incontinence appliances	q
Signs/symptoms/ill defined (D)	R	Stoma appliances	s

Coding purity

Coding purists feel that data entered should, whenever possible, include a diagnosis. For example, if you want to record a cough, you should only do it as a symptom if you can't put in a diagnosis code too. For example 171. is the symptom code for cough (from Chapter 1). The diagnosis code for this patient could be H060. for acute bronchitis (from Chapter H for respiratory diseases) or B221 malignant neoplasm of the main bronchus (from Chapter B for neoplasms). The problem with just coding coughs is that one would rarely do a search for coughs (because of the number of different causes of a cough). It doesn't record enough detail. It is acceptable in the individual patient's record but less useful when auditing, researching or reporting, which is the main reason you are bothering to put the codes in at all. So for this reason some people advocate *always trying to enter a diagnosis code*, even if it is vague, like acute upper respiratory tract infection (H05z. in 5-byte Read 2). Read 2 does not help with this purist approach. Finding an appropriate diagnosis code for mild depression is not easy. All the diagnosis codes are a bit nebulous and all the useful codes are in the symptom or history chapters. These latter codes do not give much idea about how bad the patient is (*see* below). Version 3 promises to improve this but it probably serves to remind us that recording information in this rigid way reduces the ability to communicate the individual's problem and often free text is essential.

Diagnostic terms	Symptom and history terms
Brief depressive reaction	Depressed
Prolonged depressive reaction	Stress-related problem
Acute reaction to stress	Agitated
Grief reaction	H/O anxiety state
Neurotic depression reactive type	Family bereavement

New codes

There is an arrangement for each computer system supplier to pass requests for any particular codes up to the company who run the Read code distribution, who will often implement them six months or so later.

Finding codes

The most frustrating thing about GP computers for many new users is the time they spend searching through a long list of confusing possibilities for the code that describes what they want. Usually it is not necessary or useful to type the whole of a word you want to search for. For instance typing Kellers will draw a blank, whereas Keller will find Keller's osteotomy, synonym KELLER. Never type more than ten letters, because the abbreviated forms are only ten letters long.

Some codes in version 2 for common, important (and one bizarre) events and given below. At the bottom are some useful codes to use when you can't find a really descriptive one:

Abbreviation (not guaranteed)		5-byte	4-byte
Esse	For essential hypertension	G20	G31.
Hyperten	For all hypertensive disease	G2...	G3.
Asthma	For all asthma	H33..	H43.
Diabet	For all diabetes	C10	C2..
ante or pregnan	For antenatal care	62...	62..
urti	For URTI	H05z.	H1..
MED3	For the sick certificates	9D11	9D11
MED5	For more certificates	9D21	9D21
check	A list of lots of checks	Very useful	Less useful
DNA	Did not attend	9N42	9N42.
Smoking	Health ed – smoking (advised to stop)	6791	6791

cont.

Abbreviation (not guaranteed)		5-byte	4-byte
BP	O/E BP reading (enables recording the reading)	246..	246.
repeat	Repeated prescription	8B41.	84B1
spacec	Spacecraft accident NOS, member of ground crew injured	T55z1	Less specific!
Locum	Seen by locum doctor	9N2D.	9N2D
GP su	Seen in GP's surgery	9N11.	9N11
home v	Home visit	9N1C.	9N1C
chat	Had a chat to patient (aim to use rarely)	8CB..	8CB.
Advice g	Advice about treatment given	677B.	67BB
Usual	Usual warning given	8CD..	8CD
Drug	Drug therapy NOS	8B3Z.	8B3Z

Some practices have set up their own abbreviations that limit the diagnoses codes that are initially given. For example, LBP for low back pain may give just the five most common causes of pain rather than all the causes of back pain. This makes selection of codes within a practice more consistent and subsequent reporting more accurate.

Important notes

Abbreviations and other cryptic notes in the Read codes

NOS stands for not otherwise specified.

NEC stands for not elsewhere classified.

EC stands for elsewhere classified (as in 'other event EC').

[D] means a 'vague' symptom used as a working diagnosis (i.e. half of GP consultations, headache, abdominal pain, etc.).

[SO] means 'site of' intended operation but is often used as symptom(s) (of).

[V] means it is one of the terms the UK added to the ICD-9 classification (yes of course we adopted the international standard ... with just a few changes. They are revealingly called 'The V terms'.

[M] terms are morphology terms, mainly of cancer. Don't use them unless you have a pathology report and have noted where the tumour is.

F/H means family history (this is not a diagnosis code).

H/O means history of (this is not a diagnosis code).

Ways to code

Natural language

Typing in the first few letters of term required

Hypert	Many matches
Hypertension	19 matches
Ess hyp	6 matches
Mal ess hyp	1 match

Use key words, first three letters, abbreviations (CVA, BP, BMI), lay terms, sites, eponyms (Parkinson's, Alzheimer's).
Avoid Acute, chronic, disease, hyper, hypo.

Direct code entry

Entering the code itself.

Browsing

Searching the codes by moving up and down the hierarchy.

G   Circulatory disease
    G3   Ischaemic heart disease
        G30   Acute myocardial infarction
            G301   Anterior myocardial infarction
                G3011   Acute anteroseptal myocardial infarction

However, hierarchies are not always logical....
Try looking for 'fibroids'.

Female pelvic inflammatory diseases	K4...
Other female genital tract diseases	K5...

Neoplasms	B....
Benign neoplasms	B7...
Fibroids	B78..

Computer generated

Computer selected according to protocols or templates.

Exercises

Exercise 1: Patient's notes

How would you code the following extract from a patient's notes?

3/8/98	Home Visit C/o chest pain, central tight, SOB at rest O/E BP 100/60 P98 AF, HS NAD basal creps Δ MI admit CCU stat Aspirin 150mg given
10/8/98	Discharged from hospital 8/8/98 Dyspepsia On ranitidine 150mg BD Awaiting OPD for endoscopy/Hypylori tests
24/9/98	Endoscopy – Reflux, Hpylori neg Asymptomatic now BP 120/70 P82AF for ECG smokes 15d leaflet given Rx Ranitidine 150mg
27/9/98	Nurse Clinic – ECG done
28/9/98	ECG – AF advised Aspirin 150mg daily

Exercise 2: terms to try

Term	Code
O/E grossly enlarged tonsils	
FBC	
TURP	
X-ray soft tissue chest wall	
Med 3 issued	
Bronchoscopy	
Uterine fibroids	
Gout	
Anaemia – iron deficiency	
MS	
Chronic duodenal ulcer with perforation	
Nappy rash	
FB in ear	
Contraceptive counselling	
UTI post-op	
Orthopaedic referral	
Cold sore	

Term	Code
Patient pregnant	
Occupation – GP	
Cholesterol screen	
DVT leg	
Asthma	
F/H Asthma	
Closed fracture clavicle	
H/O ectopic pregnancy	
Cauterisation of interna nose	

Answers

Exercise 1: Patient's notes

3/8/98	Home Visit **9N1C** C/o chest pain **1822** central tight, SOB at rest **1734** O/E BP 100/60 **246 &** **Reading** P98 AF **G5730**, HS NAD **24B1** basal creps **23D** Δ MI **G30** admit CCU **8H2** stat Aspirin 150mg given **bu25**
10/8/98	**9N11** (GP Surgery) Discharged from hospital 8/8/98 Dyspepsia **J16y4** On ranitidine 150mg BD Awaiting OPD for endoscopy/Hypylori tests **9R56**
24/9/98	Endoscopy – Reflux **J10y4**, Hpylori neg **4JO1** Asymptomatic now BP 120/70 **246 & Reading** P82 AF **G5730** for ECG **3211** smokes 15d **1374** leaflet given **6791** Rx Ranitidine 150mg **a628/a62v**
27/9/98	Nurse Clinic **9N22** – ECG done **321**
28/9/98	ECG **3272** – AF advised Aspirin 150mg daily **8CA3 8BC3**

Exercise 2: terms to try

Term	Code
O/E grossly enlarged tonsils	2DB4
FBC	424
TURP	7B390
X-ray soft tissue chest wall	5365
Med 3 issued	9D11
Bronchoscopy	744Bz
Uterine fibroids	B78
Gout	C34
Anaemia – iron deficiency	D00
MS	F20
Chronic duodenal ulcer with perforation	J1212
Nappy rash	M110
FB in ear	SG1
Contraceptive counselling	6777
UTI post-op	K1902
Orthopaedic referral	8H54
Cold sore	2524
Patient pregnant	62
Occupation – GP	03DC
Cholesterol screen	6879
DVT leg	G8015
Asthma	H33
F/H Asthma	12D2
Closed fracture clavicle	S200
H/O ectopic pregnancy	1544
Cauterisation of interna nose	74040

Acknowledgements

This brief synopsis of Read codes has been developed based on a combination of three documents and the author's own experiences.[36–38]

Appendix 13
North Cumbria PRIMIS case study: at the heart of good practice

In September 1999, the North Cumbria Health Authority began work on a project designed to help its GPs record good quality patient data on their clinical computer systems, with the primary objective of supporting patient care. This case study charts the course of the project during its first 18 months, highlighting the lessons learned and the supporting role played by primary care information services (PRIMIS) in getting the project up and running.

The background

Dr Rob Walker, Director, Primary and Community Care
'We first had the idea seven or eight years ago of trying to capture quality data, but we were really hamstrung by the lack of computing development at practice level, and the logistic difficulties of getting people to record simple data in a really consistent way. And so it went into the pending tray, until the computerisation of practices improved and we got to the stage where something like PRIMIS could come in.'

'Two factors have helped us to get to where we are today. Firstly, we have a long track record of trying to make data meaningful. We developed a system in-house which allowed us to use data and feed it back to practices in a comparative way, which caused an enormous amount of interest because, for the very first time in general practice, people could see their work had relevance. The actual recording of the data became less of a chore because they realised it wasn't going to just disappear into some black hole. Secondly, as a health authority, we had a good relationship with GPs, and we understood that you couldn't simply go along to busy practices and expect them to do all this extra work without giving them some tangible help.'

Planning the project

David Foster, Head of Information
'Our interest in PRIMIS was first prompted by national service frameworks (NSFs), *Information for Health*, electronic patient records (EPRs), and the move towards paperless practices, all of which suggested that the use of clinical systems within practices needed to be encouraged. We had known for a number of years that the use of practice systems was haphazard in terms of the quality and coverage of clinical data collected: some practices were keen to forge ahead, others used their systems sparingly. This meant that data collected for morbidity studies, for example, was – at best – difficult. In September 1999, a small amount of *Information for Health* money was made available to employ a PRIMIS facilitator, whose role would be to look at how data could be collected within practices to support patient care electronically and which, in the longer term, will be used in morbidity studies within the primary care groups and local health authority.'

Relevant data

'An action plan was developed which emphasised the primary objective of collecting quality health data to the benefit of patient care, and this plan gave a broad outline to the North Cumbria Clinical Governance Steering Group, which was overseeing the project. We visited other PRIMIS schemes in Northumberland and Lancashire to get some background knowledge of what was involved, and a visit to a GP practice did a lot to set the scene for the project in North Cumbria. The main message we received from that practice was that if data is to be collected, it has to be data that is relevant to the doctor/patient relationship; that will help the doctor in the care of that patient; and that the doctor can collect quite easily – because the last thing he or she wants is to be looking through a massive Read code book. Another clear message was that data needs to be recorded in a consistent manner.'

Quality data

'A very important principle for us was to avoid running before we could walk. Although some felt that we should extract data immediately and see what it was telling us, we knew that that would be a pointless exercise unless it was good quality data. So we decided not to run in and do data extraction from the outset, but to start slowly and methodically, and to learn in some detail from a first wave of practices what exactly would be required of us ... what the real problems and issues were. We have three primary care groups (PCGs) in North Cumbria covering 320 000 patients in 56 practices, and we decided to do the project in several phases.'

'Our first objective was to record good quality information, and we believe this is best done if the data collected supports the consultation between practice staff and their patients. In this way, high quality data will then be available, as a by-product, to support a range of activities, such as morbidity studies and practice audit.'

Relationship to local implementation strategy for information for health

'*Information for Health* recognised the strategic importance of EPRs and EHRs. A wide-ranging board, consisting of clinical and managerial members, considered PRIMIS (CHDGP as it was then) to be a significant piece of work which would help to deliver the EPR in a primary care setting, and also offer a rich source of data which could be used in needs assessment to support the local development of strategies and plans. Clinical governance and NSFs have served to increase the importance of the work undertaken. PRIMIS is now a significant element of the LIS in taking forward the various agendas within North Cumbria.'

Getting started – the pilot stage

Carol Smith, Project Manager (formerly PRIMIS facilitator)
'Having done our research, prepared the project plan and data collection agreement, and received our initial training from PRIMIS, we decided to do a pilot study in order to understand what practices expected from the project, and to define what data was to be collected. Eight practices who were known to be recording data took part in this pilot. They were drawn from all three PCGs in North Cumbria and varied in size and type, ranging from a small remote practice with two GPs, to a large inner city practice with eight GPs. They used a variety of clinical systems – EMIS, Vision, Vamp Medical and Meditel. During this pilot stage, I

spent two days with each practice, speaking to one or more of the GPs, the practice manager, practice nurses and other staff.'

Feedback

'All the practices which took part in the pilot were very positive and as a result, all eight wanted to move on and become "First Wave" PRIMIS practices in the North Cumbria project. They all seemed aware of the importance of standardised data both within and across practices. The pilot practices were all different in terms of how they were currently operating with regard to electronic data recording and coding. For example, in one practice, one GP records and codes all consultation data on the system, whereas another GP in the practice never switches the computer on, and the remaining GPs record data at differing levels in between. We soon realised that different practices and practice staff would need different levels of assistance, support and encouragement.'

Templates

'Many of the messages from the pilot study were what we were expecting. One was that if doctors were to collect data, it needed to be in a simple way. Another strong message was that templates were needed to capture data in a standard way; some EMIS practices were already using default templates. Participants agreed on the importance of developing templates to meet both practice needs in supporting patient care, and to fulfil the agreed North Cumbria data sets. It was agreed that, as the facilitator, I would work with each practice to design templates for the four priority disease areas, which had been identified, namely coronary heart disease, (CHD), hypertension, asthma and diabetes. Minimum data sets were agreed upon for all practices during the pilot stage, training needs were identified, and a schedule was drawn up. Most of the practices had no template skills in-house and I would, therefore, develop their templates for them. One practice already had template design skills in-house and I would work alongside them to ensure compliance with the core data set and coding consistencies across practices.'

Issues of concern

'Many of the practices raised time as an issue of concern. It was pointed out that since the practices were already recording consultation data electronically, the project would not take up more time and, in fact, would save time once templates had been introduced. It was agreed, however, that if the current data quality was found to be poor after the first data quality extraction, additional time would be needed to improve data quality. Time would also have to be set aside for staff training. Training needs were identified as:

- the use of templates
- Read code structure
- skills in 'using' data – i.e. extracting, presenting and analysing
- designing templates.

Using templates and the Read code structure would need to be tackled at an early stage, but skills in using data and template design were skills that were not so urgent and these could be undertaken at a later date. Some GPs were identified as needing additional training, and time would be spent with them to encourage them to record data.'

The North Cumbria PRIMIS project in action: an overview of the first 18 months

September 1999	• PRIMIS Facilitator recruited • Presentation by PRIMIS Service Director, Sheila Teasdale, to clinical governance group
October 1999	• Visit to Nottingham to meet PRIMIS team • Research visits to two PRIMIS schemes
November 1999	• Production of project plan • Facilitator training by PRIMIS: training needs assessment/data quality/Read code • Research visits to two health authorities and one GP practice (PRIMIS participants)
December 1999	• Further development of project plan
January 2000	• Practices invited to take part in pilot study • Preparatory work for pilot study
February 2000 March 2000	• Pilot study undertaken in eight practices
April 2000	• Findings of pilot study reported and agreement reached on the way forward for the North Cumbria PRIMIS project • Facilitator training by PRIMIS: MIQUEST • Facilitator training by system suppliers: EMIS, In Practice and Meditel

May 2000	• MIQUEST set up and data quality queries run in eight first wave practices • Visits to practices to assess template and training needs; production of training timetable
June 2000 July 2000	• Implementation of PRIMIS and training in practices (one week spent in each)
August 2000	• Follow-up visits to practices • Research and development – EMIS protocols set up • Invitations sent out for second wave PRIMIS
September 2000	• Confirmation of eight second wave PRIMIS practices • Vision templates set up for electronic referrals in area of colorectal cancer • Second MIQUEST extraction at first wave practices • Facilitator training by PRIMIS: data quality feedback
October 2000	• Research in eight second wave PRIMIS practices • MIQUEST set up and data quality queries run in eight second wave practices • Second MIQUEST extraction in first wave practices
November 2000	• Preparatory work at second wave practices • CHD queries run in first wave practices • Feedback of data quality analysis to first wave practices • First wave practices trained to run MIQUEST queries
December 2000 January 2001 February 2001	• Third MIQUEST extraction in first wave practices • Implementation of PRIMIS and training in second wave practices (one week spent in each) • Recruitment of two new facilitators

The North Cumbria PRIMIS project in practice

Dr Mark Taylor, GP

'PRIMIS came at exactly the right time for us. We had computerised in 1991, and by 1992 our notes were fully summarised and organised with a repeat prescribing system, which we thought was almost foolproof. We ran with that for five years, but then changed from a Vamp system to EMIS – and promptly lost 5%

of our data! The prescribing data, which had gone onto a back screen, had to be brought back and rejigged into the EMIS system. Then there were one or two diagnoses where the Read codes didn't match and therefore it didn't transfer properly. It was then we realised that Read codes were probably quite important, because if we had Read coded all our data on the Vamp system, most of it would have transferred directly to where we wanted it on the EMIS system. But we didn't – we ran our own little system, we invented a few codes of our own, which we've now suffered from because, of course, we had to redo them – for smoking, in particular.'

'The system now runs very well and our clinics are all computer-based. We are actually 85% paperless now and are all using the computer in our consultations, which we were not doing a year ago. The nurses have started to use the computer and our health visitors are putting vaccinations on to the computer, so we are getting everyone used to the fact that it is a computer-led service now.'

Disease management

'We had started to look at our chronic disease management and were thinking about the fact that we had to set up templates, when Carole came along with the PRIMIS project. It picked up on things we were particularly interested in. Diabetes is our target focus this year in clinical governance, and this system is absolutely perfect. It means you can access the data very easily and audit it very simply. The diabetic audit used to be a couple of days' work to put it all together, but now it will take about half an hour to get the data. CHD at NSF level is the one we're delivering with public health at the moment in the PCG; so again, it is providing a framework on diseases that we are very keen to develop. We have set up a cardio rehab clinic with a template, calling in all our angina and heart attack patients by rote, using the cardio rehab template and its recall date to actually manage their care.'

'We now have an asthma template, which is user-friendly and serves two functions: it supplies the data that the health authority would like to collect, and it also gives the practice what it wants as well. The asthma template is a very dynamic one, because we are using it to take people off the register. We had a lot of asthmatics on our database who are not asthmatic any more because they had it when they were young and are now better. So the template is useful for screening out that sort of data. This meant that when we identified patients on prophylactic asthma treatment during our asthma audit, the numbers had decreased and we wondered where we had gone wrong. In fact, what had happened was that we had actually contracted the asthma base. It makes data collecting a lot more complicated. It means you have to be up to date because asthma data is dynamic and changing all the time. We have also changed our system, with the asthma clinic now being by invitation, rather than by appointment. This means that the template becomes even more important, to identify who the defaulters are who do not attend. We then decide if we really do need to see those patients or not, based on the condition of their asthma, and we chase them if necessary.'

Problems

'Every GP is an individual and there are GPs that are interested in computers, and others who do not like them and believe they take away from direct patient contact and patient care. So, in a practice of eight partners, you might get four who are really enthusiastic, two who will go along with it, and two who won't turn their computers on. So, immediately, your data is in trouble because a quarter of it doesn't exist – it is still in the notes. Making data recording as simple as possible is very important. Making it as user-friendly as possible is also important.'

Using templates

'Nurses are wonderful at using templates and will go through them individually in detail. It also helps that they are collecting data, which we do use. For example, diabetes is shared care – it is not GP care. It is very important for audit to know what has happened to our diabetics and the template takes you into it straight away. The discipline is to work through the template from the top to the bottom and not to jump it because you are busy. You find that if you are doing a cardio rehab clinic or a diabetic clinic, you take time to go into the template and work your way through it. If you are in the middle of a busy morning surgery and someone comes in ten minutes late for a blood pressure check, it is very easy to take the blood pressure, do the prescription and let them go, without using the template because you are aware of the fact that you are pushed for time and things are busy. You have to be quite disciplined to use a template.'

The benefits

'I think that PRIMIS has come at the right time for primary care – as PCGs become PCTs and as information technology is developing rapidly. We needed something like this to gear it all up and drive the agenda out to practices. The big advantage of PRIMIS is that it can go to all the PCGs, so we can be certain that they are moving in the same direction, collecting data of the same quality, and in the same way.

'PRIMIS has speeded things up and has done it in a much more organised way. Carol met with all the people who were meant to be using the information and explained to them individually how the system would work, which was very helpful to us. And because Carol developed the templates and knew all about them, she knew what the quirks were as well, so that she could answer all the queries the staff had. All the staff got the same level of training and were not just told what they ought to do. I think that was particularly important. It was done quickly and effectively, because sometimes these things take months to implement, and by the time you get everyone trained, those who were trained first have forgotten much of it! Carol just came and lived in the practice for a week, which was ideal. We have our own internal training programmes but we would have found it very hard to give that kind of input.'

The results so far

Initial results from the First Wave of practices suggest that templates appear to have improved data quality in:

- identifying additional patients with CHD, hypertension, asthma or diabetes
- significantly improving the associated lifestyle data being recorded for patients with CHD, hypertension, asthma or diabetes.

A baseline extraction of data quality and CHD data was undertaken at practices prior to implementation. Subsequent extractions have been carried out at three-monthly intervals following implementation, to track progress.

Figures 1 and 2 show recording improvements in four of the practices after the introduction of templates and necessary training.

The attitude of practices has been positive, with staff viewing the project as supporting them in patient care and in the use of their clinical systems, rather than as something imposed on them by the health authority. Practice staff are more

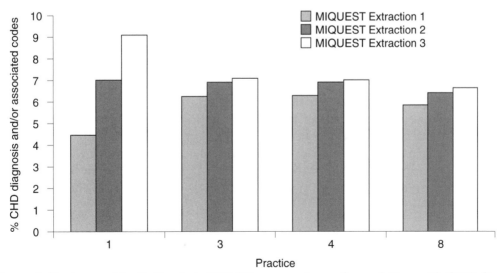

Figure 1: First wave North Cumbria PRIMIS – percentage of population with CHD diagnosis and/or CHD-associated codes.

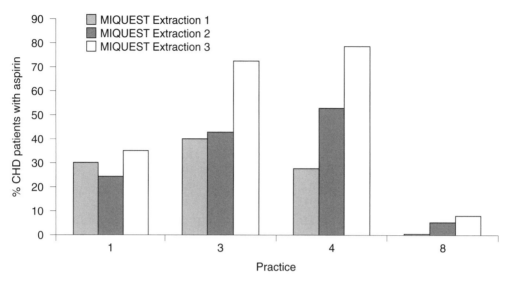

Figure 2: First wave North Cumbria PRIMIS – percentage of CHD patients with aspirin recorded.

willing to use their clinical system, and the project is seen as a good way of collecting data to support other agendas, such as NSF performance monitoring.

The future of the North Cumbria PRIMIS Project

In August 2000, an invitation was sent out to every practice manager and GP in North Cumbria to recruit practices for the second wave. Responses came back within a week, and not only was the second wave fully signed up, but practices were placed on a waiting list for the third wave.

It had become obvious during the pilot stage that the resource implications of North Cumbria's approach had been underestimated and that to move the project forward in the desired manner, one facilitator per 20 practices would be needed. Additional funding was, therefore, found for the recruitment of two new facilitators, which would enable the project to be rolled out more effectively and quickly.

Future plans involve:

- the complete roll-out of PRIMIS in the four priority clinical areas
- similar work in new clinical areas (such as cancer and mental health)
- gaining sufficient expertise in Read codes for the facilitators to be able to offer advice and support to practices in North Cumbria

- providing a comprehensive service to practices in examining and improving their data quality, leading to the establishment of a morbidity database containing quality data
- offering practices guidance and support regarding template development, particularly on coding issues
- promoting the use of information within practices and providing the necessary training to support this process.

In addition to the above priorities, the team in North Cumbria will continue to support existing PRIMIS practices. This will include continuously working on data quality, providing analysis and feedback, running MIQUEST queries, maintaining the PRIMIS database at the health authority, acting as a help desk facility, undertaking revisions to templates as necessary, and – in cases where practices change their computer system – working with the practices concerned to develop templates on their new system and provide the appropriate training.

Those involved are enthusiastic about the future of the project.

The project manager's perspective: Carol Smith
'With the resource of two additional facilitators, we should be able to offer all practices in North Cumbria the same level of service that has been offered to the ones who have already participated, with complete coverage of all 56 practices by March 2002.'

'We learnt during the pilot study that the MIQUEST compliance of certain systems is not as good as some suppliers claim, so we have limited ourselves in the second wave to practices with particular clinical systems. This also enables us to manage the time better, as we will be concentrating on fewer systems which will free up time to devote to more analytical and data quality work.'

'As part of the pilot study we have identified the need to produce a North Cumbria PRIMIS Read directory to include Read codes and terms for everyday consultations/problems/encounters (for example, flu, backache, migraine. The suggestions of all the GPs in the scheme will be brought together, appropriate codes allocated to problems, and two directories produced (4-byte Read and version 2 Read), to be distributed to all clinical staff involved in the project. This will assist clinical staff to record everyday consultation data and will begin to set standards in all areas of health care. A fuller, more detailed directory could be developed in the future.'

'At present we have a waiting list for North Cumbria PRIMIS, and practices are coming forward expressing their interest in joining the scheme: in effect, North Cumbria PRIMIS is selling itself.'

The health authority perspective: Dr Rob Walker
'I think that we are going to have real hard morbidity data from primary care. To me, it is a goldmine of information to actually see where resources are going to be

needed in the future, and it is going to be real hard data, not "top of the head" stuff. We will also be able to get really accurate information about the prevalence of disease and how it is managed. Regular audit and self-assessment of standards of care is very difficult without the data. Every time you wanted to audit a particular condition, you would have to set up a special project to collect morbidity data. Now you just press a button and it should be there.'

'We did say at the outset that we should take our time with this project, and it has been a very painstaking process. But I think it is going to pay off. One of our PCGs, which covers about 20 practices, has now taken the decision to try and commit every one to the PRIMIS programme, which is quite a step forward. We have a lot of support from the three PCGs who, I believe, see the PRIMIS system as an aid to their management in the future. The whole process of setting up the PRIMIS process has improved the relationship between the health authority and its constituent practices, and the value of that should not be underestimated.'

The GP perspective: Dr Mark Taylor

'I think, as things develop, we will need the input of the PRIMIS facilitator to develop new templates and new services. It is useful to have ongoing data extractions because that tells you how you are getting on. If your data quality starts to slip, it warns you that you need to be sorting it out again. It is important that, as new doctors and nurses come into the practice, we have a comprehensive training programme.'

'This is a great research tool, which we could actually use in the future as part of research and development. The PRIMIS facilitator's expertise could be used to set up a template to do a research project with maybe a dozen practices taking part, which would be quality data for a quality project. As computer systems become more advanced and more developed, I believe templates will be used more and more.'

Highlights from the North Cumbria PRIMIS project

- Pre-project research.
- Clear objectives.
- Planning in phases.
- Realistic targets.
- Building of relationships.
- Facilitator training and support for practice staff.
- Simple, relevant and consistent data recording.

- Importance of templates.
- Quality data in support of patient care.

Source: Reproduced with permission from PRIMIS (2001) *North Cumbria: at the heart of good practice, Case study*. PRIMIS, Nottingham. http://www.primis.nottingham.ac.uk[35]

Glossary

ACORN	CACI's geodemographic consumer targeting classification
BMA	British Medical Association
BNF	*British National Formulary*
CACI	Company specialising in market analysis, information systems and direct marketing
CHDGP	Collection of Health Data from General Practice
CME	Continuing medical education
Commissioning	Replacement for fundholding. GPs and other healthcare providers decide best healthcare for their patients
CPD	Continuing professional development
CPT	Current procedural terminology
CSM	Committee on Safety of Medicines
DIN	Doctors independent network
DoH	Department of Health (UK)
eBNF	electronic *British National formulary*
EDI	Electronic data interchange
EDIFACT	Electronic data interchange for administration, commerce and transport
EHR	Electronic health record
EPR	Electronic patient record
FHSA	Family health service authority
Fundholding	Scheme whereby GPs control their own budget to decide the best healthcare for their patients
GMC	General Medical Council

GMS	General medical services. Services a GP is expected to provide on the NHS
GP	General practice/practitioner
GPnet	General Practice Network programme
HA	Health authority. Managerial level of the NHS concerned with co-ordinating healthcare provision (England and Wales)
HQL	Health query language
ICD	International classification of diseases
ICT	Information communication technologies
IM&T	Information management and technology
IMG	Information management group
Independent/ contractor status	Term which refers to the self-employed status of GPs while still being an integral part of the NHS
IT	Information technology
IOS	Items of service. Includes claims for: night visits, treatment of a temporary resident, registration of a new patient, immediate necessary treatment, child health surveillance, contraceptive services, maternity medical services, vaccination and immunisation, minor surgery
JCPTGP	Joint Committee of Postgraduate Training for General Practice
LIS	Local implementation strategy
MCA	Medicines Control Agency
Micros	Microcomputers
MIQUEST	Morbidity Information Query Export SynTax
MSIA	Medical Software Industry Association
NAS	New active substance
NeLH	National electronic Library for Health
NHS	National Health Service
NHS CCC	National Health Service Centre for Coding and Classification
NHSE	National Health Service Executive
NHSIA	National Health Service Information Authority
NHSnet	National Health Service network
NICE	National Institute for Clinical Excellence
Non-principal	A practitioner not contracted with a health authority to take unsupervised responsibility for patients
NSF	National Service Framework
OOH	Out of hours. Periods outside the 'normal' working hours of 9am–7pm Monday to Friday, 8am–1pm Saturdays
OPCS	Office of Population, Censuses and Surveys
OPCS4	Office of Population Censuses and Surveys classification of surgical operations and procedures
PACT	Prescribing Analysis and CosT
PC	Personal computer

PCC	Primary care centres
PCG	Primary care group
PCO	Primary care organisation
PCT	Primary care trust
PGEA	Postgraduate education allowance
PPA	Prescription Pricing Authority
PRESTIGE	Patient REcords Supporting TelematIcs and GuidelinEs
Primary care	The first level of healthcare normally accessed by patients (e.g. general practitioners, dentists, opticians)
Primary care team	The clinicians or healthcare professionals in a general practice, together with the administration team (practice manager, data entry and record personnel, etc.)
PRIMIS	Primary care information services
Principal	A practitioner who is contracted to take unsupervised responsibility for patients
PRODIGY	Prescribing RatiOnally with Decision support In General practice studY
Protocols	A written statement of procedures
R&D	Research and Development
RCGP	Royal College of General Practitioners (UK)
Red Book	Properly known as *The Statement of Fees and Allowances*, outlines GPs' pay from providing GMS
RFA	Requirements for accreditation
RFP	Request for a proposal
RHA	Regional health authority
SBO	State-based organisation
Secondary Care	Second level of healthcare normally accessed by patients (e.g. hospitals), usually referred from GPs and others in primary care
SNOMED	Systemised Nomenclature of Medicine – a classification system for medicine
Template	A template is a data entry screen on a general practice computer system which has been constructed so as to prompt the user to record certain items which arise in certain clinical situations, such as chronic disease monitoring, new patient registration, 'well person' clinics, etc. As well as providing a prompt for the information, a template should also ensure that the correct code is entered into the patient's record
Tertiary care	The third level of healthcare normally accessed by patients – highly specialised treatment centres often located in larger hospitals
TSSA	Transplant Support Service Authority
UKTSSA	United Kingdom Transplant Support Service Authority
UPS	Uninterruptible power supply

References

1 Fogarty L (1997) Primary care informatics development: one view through the miasma. *Journal of Informatics in Primary Care*. **January:** 2–11.
2 Department of Health (1997) *The New NHS: modern, dependable*. DoH, London.
3 NHSE (1998) *Information for Health: an information strategy for the modern NHS 1998–2005*. NHSE, London.
4 General Medical Council's General Practitioners' Committee and the Royal College of General Practitioners on behalf of the NHS Executive (2000) *Good Practice Guidelines for General Practice Electronic Patient Records*. GMC, London. http://www.doh.gov.uk/gpepr/index.html
5 NHSE (2001) *Building the Information Core: implementing the NHS Plan*. NHSE, Leeds.
6 RFA http://nhsia.nhs.uk/rfa.frhome.html
7 MIQUEST http://www.clinical-info.co.uk/miquest.htm
8 NHSE (1998) *Evaluation of GP Computer Systems 1997: national report*. NHSE, London.
9 NHSE (1998) *Evaluation of GP Computer Systems 1997: national report*. General Practice Systems Accreditation (E5409). NHSE, Leeds.
10 GPCG (1999) Request for a proposal (RFP). In: GPCG *Buying Computer Systems For General Practice*. Version 1.1, June.
11 GPCG (1999) Contract checklist. In: GPCG *Buying Computer Systems For General Practice*. Version 1.1, June.
12 DoH (1999) *Electronic Patient Records Move a Step Closer: NHS and College of American Pathologists to create world standard in clinical terminology*. Press release, 14 April: reference 1999/0232.
13 http://www.doh.gov.uk/hshipmanpractice
14 DoH (2000) *Electronic patient medical records in primary care: changes to the GP terms of service*. (Letter from Mike Farrar including annex of guidance to Health Authority Chief Executives, Directors of Primary Care, NHS Regional Directors, all general practices,

Chief Executives of Primary Care Trusts, Primary Care Groups and Local Medical Committees.)

15 Section 3.2, Standards. In: *Collection of Health Data from General Practice (CHDGP) Guidelines* (2000). NHS Information Authority, Exeter. http://www.nottingham.ac.uk/chdgp/

16 Applebee K (2001) 26 weeks to using computers in GP and practice nurse consultations. In: *NHS HIS Lambeth, Southwark and Lewisham Noteless Practice Support Pack: a resource for GP practices.* NHS HIS, London.

17 Gillies AC, Ellis B, Lowe N (2002) *Building an Electronic Disease Register: getting the computers to work for you.* Radcliffe Medical Press, Oxford.

18 Section 5.3, Direct data entry. In: *Collection of Health Data from General Practice (CHDGP) Guidelines* (2000). NHS Information Authority, Exeter. http://www.nottingham.ac.uk/chdgp/

19 Section 5.4, In-direct data entry. In: *Collection of Health Data from General Practice (CHDGP) Guidelines* (2000). NHS Information Authority, Exeter. http://www.nottingham.ac.uk/chdgp/

20 Gillies AC (1999) *IT and Information for Healthcare.* Radcliffe Medical Press, Oxford.

21 Gillies AC (2001) *Excel for Clinical Governance.* Radcliffe Medical Press, Oxford.

22 NHS HIS Lambeth, Southwark and Lewisham (2001) *Noteless practice support pack: a resource for GP practice.* NHS HIS, London.

23 Benson T and Neame R (1994) *Healthcare Computing.* Longman Group, Harlow.

24 Hunt D, Haynes R, Hanna S and Smith K (1998) Effects of computer-based clinical decision support systems on physician performance and patient outcomes: a systematic review. *JAMA.* **280**: 1339–46.

25 Bandolier (2000) Computer systems prevent errors. *Bandolier.* **73**: 73–5. http://www.jr2.ox.ac.uk/Bandolier/index.htm

26 Kalra D (1990) *Headings for Communicating Information for the Personal Health Record: CHIME evaluation report 2: headings within structured templates and clinical object definitions.* CHIME, UCL Medical School, London.

27 McShane M (1999) *Electronic Records and Coding.* Wisdom-pcg mailbase archives, editor. http://www.wisdom.org.uk

28 Goraya A (2000) How to switch to paperless practice. *Medical Monitor.* **46**.

29 Roscoe T (2000) Paper vs. Electronic Medical Records (Special Paper). Wisdom website: http://www.wisdom.org.uk

30 Couch J (2000) Is going paperless really cost effective? *Pulse.* **47**.

31 GPCG (1999) Buyers checklist. In: *Buying Computer Systems For General Practice.* Version 1.1, June.

32 Chelford Surgery (1999) Unpublished documentation and personal correspondence.

33 GPCG (1999) Hardware comparison checklist. In: *Buying Computer Systems For General Practice.* Version 1.1, June.

34 Rhyddings Surgery and Shadsworth Surgery (c. 2000/2001) *Beacon Information: why go paperless?*

35 PRIMIS (2001) *North Cumbria: at the heart of good practice.* Case study. PRIMIS, Nottingham. http://www.primis.nottingham.ac.uk

36 Midgley A and O'Connell S (1999) Read codes. In: *National Association of Non-Principals (NANP) Yellow Book*, Chapter 33. http://www.nanp.org.uk/index.htm

37 Torex User Group (2000) *Read Codes For Beginners*. Torex, Bromsgrove.
http://www.tmug.org.uk/index.htm
38 Tate M (2000) *Read Code Awareness Session: session notes and exercises*. PRIMIS, Nottingham.

Index